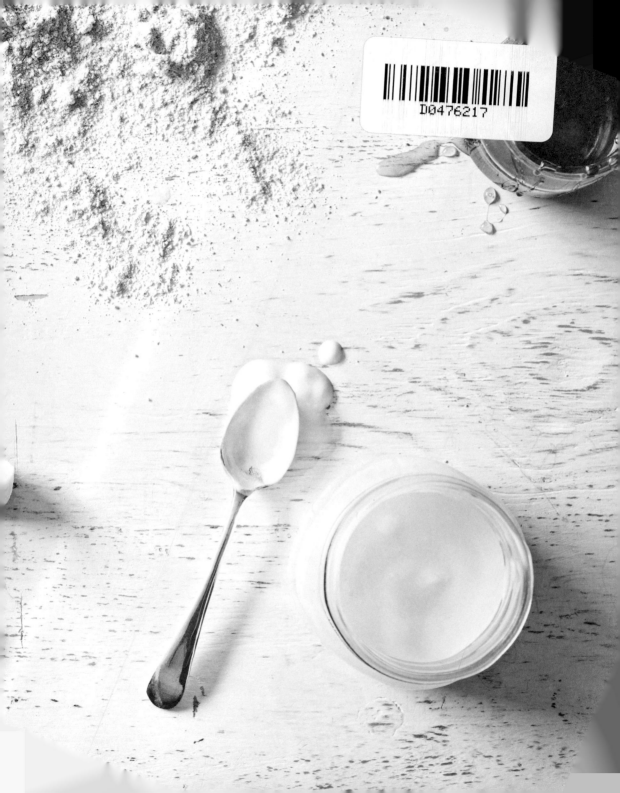

MODERN **PANCAKES**

OVER 60 CONTEMPORARY RECIPES, FROM PROTEIN PANCAKES AND HEALTHY GRAINS TO WAFFLES AND DIRTY FOOD INDULGENCES

RYLAND PETERS & SMALL
LONDON • NEW YORK

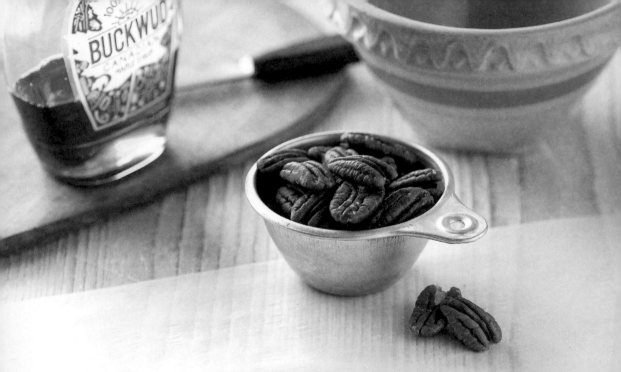

Senior Designer Toni Kay
Commissioning Editor
  Alice Sambrook
Production Controller David Hearn
Art Director Leslie Harrington
Editorial Director Julia Charles
Publisher Cindy Richards
Indexer Vanessa Bird

First published in 2019 by
Ryland Peters & Small
20–21 Jockey's Fields, London
WC1R 4BW and
341 E 116th St, New York NY 10029
www.rylandpeters.com

10 9 8 7 6 5 4 3 2

Text copyright © Amy Ruth
Finegold, Angela Romeo, Brontë
Aurell, Carol Hilker, Chloe Coker,
Dunja Gulin, Hannah Miles, Jackie
Kearney, Janet Sawyer, Jenna Zoe,
Jenny Linford, Jordan Bourke,
Kathy Kordalis, Leah Vanderveldt,
Louise Pickford, Milli Taylor,

Miranda Ballard, Rosa Rigby,
Tonia George, Valerie Aikman-
Smith, Vicky Jones. Design and
photographs copyright © Ryland
Peters & Small 2019

ISBN: 978-1-78879-068-0

Printed in China

A CIP record for this book is
available from the British Library.
US Library of Congress
Cataloging-in-Publication Data
has been applied for.

Notes:
• Both British (Metric) and American
(Imperial plus US cups) measurements
are included in these recipes for your
convenience, however it is important to
work with one set of measurements and not
alternate between the two within a recipe.
• All spoon measurements are level
unless otherwise specified.
• All eggs are medium (UK) or large (US),
unless specified as large, in which case
US extra-large should be used. Uncooked
eggs should not be served to the very old,
frail, young children, pregnant women or
those with compromised immune systems.
• Ovens should be preheated to the
specified temperatures. We recommend
using an oven thermometer. If using a
fan-assisted oven, adjust temperatures
according to the manufacturer's
instructions.
• When a recipe calls for the grated
zest of citrus fruit, buy unwaxed fruit
and wash well before using. If you can
only find treated fruit, scrub well in
warm soapy water before using.

CONTENTS

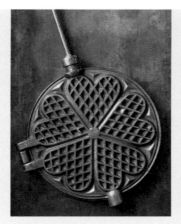

INTRODUCTION

Upgrade your pancake and waffle game with these mouth-watering recipes for the much-loved, quick and easy meal. They've always been popular tasty treats, but modern pancakes and waffles are traversing the basic breakfast boundaries of yesteryear, and breaking free to be served at breakfast, lunch and dinner tables at every occasion and to suit everyone. The beauty of pancakes and waffles is their versatility, and whether it is the ingredients in the batter, a topping, sauce or filling, the flavour variations are endless.

In the Breakfast Perfection chapter find perfect recipes for lazy Sunday mornings, indulgent brunch dishes to perk you up after a late night, and healthier pancakes with berries, oatmeal and granola to set you up right for the day.

Feeling Fruity? Recipes in this chapter are bright, zesty and full of flavour! Equally good for breakfast or dessert, try Dairy-free Coconut Pancakes with Lime Syrup & Mango, or serve the Rhubarb & Custard Crêpes for a sophisticated dessert.

What could be better than getting your five-a-day in pancake form? With a wide variety of different flours to choose from and dairy and refined sugar alternatives too, modern pancakes really can be super healthy! Turn to the Flipping Nutritious chapter to find Protein Pancakes to fuel a workout or vegan Turmeric Pancakes with Carrot Hummus & Vegetables for a virtuous yet delicious light meal.

For the more adventurous pancake eaters who think they've seen it all, the Posh Pancakes section offers exciting recipes such as Japanese Soufflé Pancakes with Coconut Cream & Passion Fruit Syrup, as well as Beetroot Pancakes with Goat's Cheese, Onion Relish & Walnuts, to serve at your next chic soirée.

If you have a sweet tooth, the Sweet & Sticky chapter will be your best friend. These filthy yet fabulous treats include Oreo Pancakes with Chocolate Fudge Sauce, Pistachio Waffles with Pistachio Ice Cream & White Chocolate Sauce and even a Red Velvet Crêpe Cake.

Finally, if you are feeling a breakfast for dinner kind of vibe, look no further than the Substantial Stacks chapter. Try Cauliflower & Chickpea Pacos with Tahini & Lime Yogurt, Pulled Pork & Cheddar Hotcakes or Spiced Green Veg Pancakes with Pineapple Chutney.

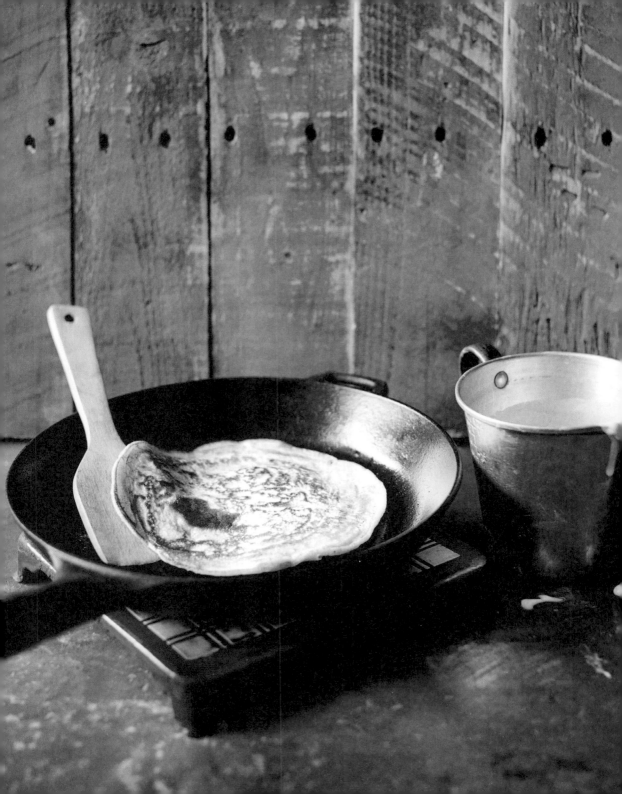

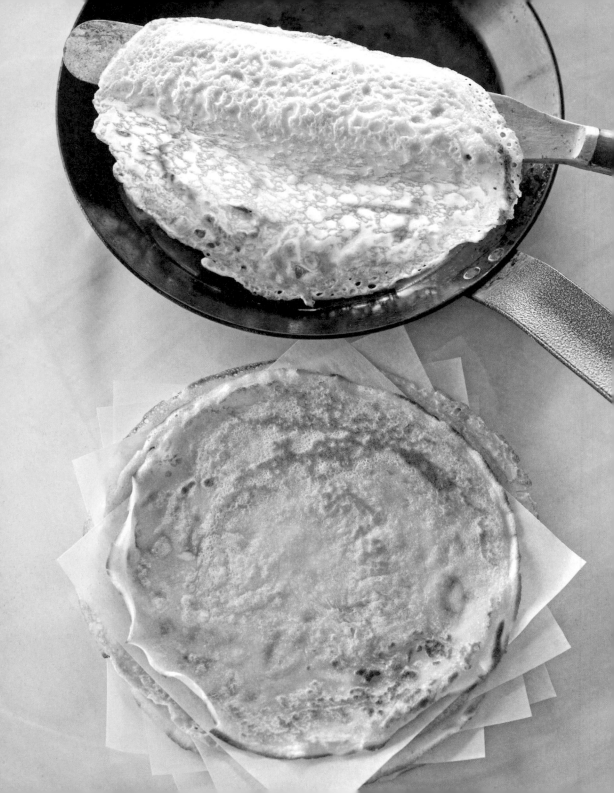

BREAKFAST PERFECTION

BAKED EGG HOPPER PANCAKES WITH TOMATO RELISH, CHORIZO & AVOCADO

Based on Indian hoppers called appams, these pancakes are made as normal and then pressed into pans to make shallow bowls for the eggs to sit in. They are then baked and served with chorizo, avocado and a smoky tomato relish.

PANCAKE BATTER

100 g/³⁄₄ cup plain/all-purpose flour

4 tablespoons chickpea (gram) flour

2 teaspoons baking powder

pinch of salt

250 ml/1 cup plus 1 tablespoon buttermilk

1 egg, beaten

FILLING

olive oil, for frying

6 eggs

1 avocado

150 g/5½ oz. chorizo, thinly sliced

50 g/scant 1 cup baby spinach

TOMATO RELISH

3 tomatoes, halved, deseeded and chopped

½ onion, finely chopped

2 tablespoons red wine vinegar

2 tablespoons dark brown sugar

¼ teaspoon smoked paprika

pinch of cayenne pepper

sea salt and freshly ground black pepper

MAKES 6

Preheat the oven to 180°C (350°F) Gas 4.

Start by making the relish. Place all the ingredients into a saucepan and season with salt and pepper. Bring to the boil and simmer, uncovered, for about 15–20 minutes, stirring occasionally, until thickened. Set aside and leave to cool.

Grease six 8 x 12 cm/3 x 5 inch pie pans with olive oil and line them with baking parchment. Set the lined pans on a large baking sheet.

To make the pancake batter, sift the plain/all-purpose flour, chickpea (gram) flour, baking powder and salt into a large mixing bowl. Make a well in the centre and beat in the buttermilk and egg to make a smooth batter.

Lightly oil a pancake pan and place over a medium heat. Once hot, add about 80 ml/⅓ cup of the batter and tilt the pan, allowing the batter to spread across in an even layer. Cook for about 2–3 minutes until the base is browned and the top set. Remove from the pan and very carefully transfer to one of the prepared pie pans, pressing it down to fit snugly inside in a bowl shape.

Repeat for the rest of the batter and pancakes (you should be able to make about six from the batter). Crack an egg into each pancake and bake in the preheated oven for 8–10 minutes until the eggs are just set.

Meanwhile, peel, destone and cut the avocado into slices and set aside. Heat a tablespoon of oil in a small frying pan/skillet over a medium heat and gently fry the chorizo slices for 2–3 minutes until golden.

Remove the baked egg hoppers from the oven and top each one with a little fried chorizo, avocado slices, spinach and a spoonful of the tomato relish. Drizzle over any chorizo cooking oil and serve.

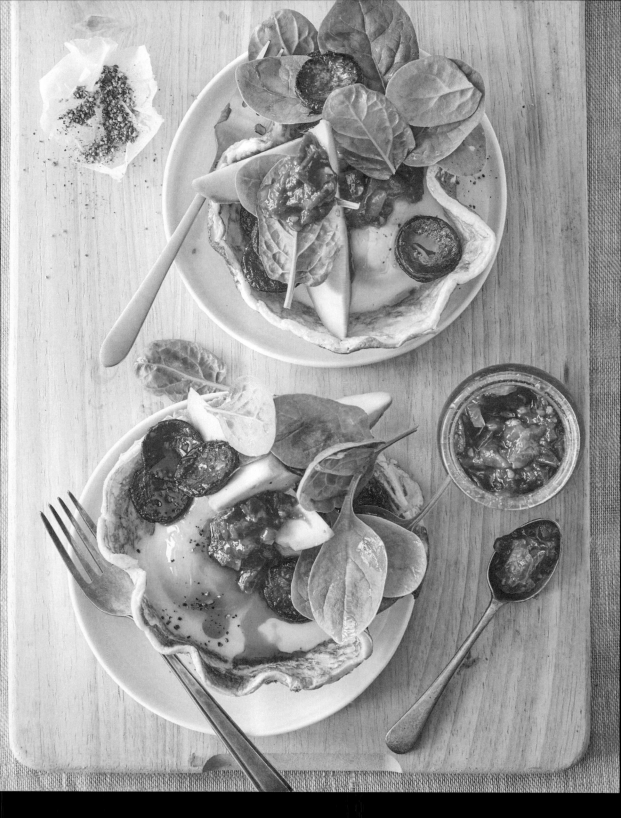

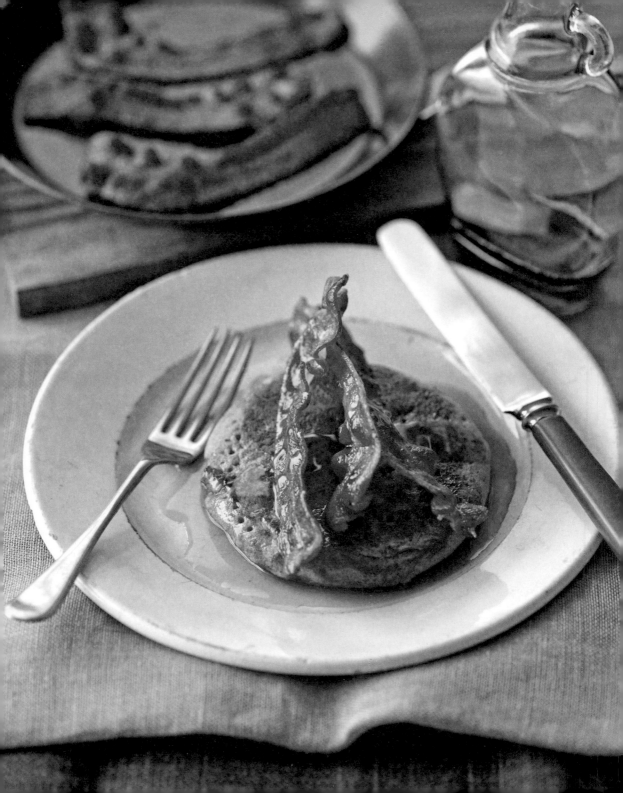

BEER & BACON PANCAKES

Beer for breakfast? Yes, you heard that right! The much-loved beverage is used here in place of milk to bind the batter. It gives the pancakes a savoury, malty flavour, which goes perfectly with salty bacon and sweet maple syrup.

PANCAKE BATTER

200 g/1½ cups smoked bacon lardons/diced pancetta

160 g/scant 1¼ cups self-raising/rising flour, sifted

1 teaspoon baking powder

1 egg, separated

60 g/⅓ cup minus 1 teaspoon dark brown sugar

pinch of salt

250 ml/1 cup plus 1 tablespoon beer

3 tablespoons melted butter, plus extra for frying

TO SERVE

12 slices of fried smoked streaky bacon/bacon strips

maple syrup

SERVES 6

Begin by frying the bacon lardons/diced pancetta in a dry frying pan/skillet – it will release sufficient oil as it cooks to prevent it sticking, so there's no need to add any extra fat to the pan. Remove the bacon from the pan and put on paper towels to let any excess fat drain. Set aside.

To make the pancake batter, put the flour, baking powder, egg yolk, dark brown sugar, salt and beer in a large mixing bowl and whisk together. Add the melted butter and whisk again. The batter should have a smooth, dropping consistency. Stir in the cooked bacon lardons/diced pancetta.

In a separate bowl, whisk the egg white to stiff peaks. Gently fold the whisked egg white into the batter mixture using a spatula. Cover and put in the refrigerator to rest for 30 minutes.

When you are ready to serve remove your batter mixture from the refrigerator and stir gently, then cook it in batches. Put a little butter in a large frying pan/skillet set over a medium heat. Allow the butter to melt and coat the base of the pan, then ladle small amounts of the rested batter into the pan, leaving a little space between each. Cook until the underside of each pancake is golden brown and a few bubbles start to appear on the top – this will take about 2–3 minutes. Turn the pancakes over using a spatula and cook on the other side until golden brown.

Serve the pancakes with extra fried streaky bacon/bacon strips and lashings of maple syrup.

MUSHROOM, BACON & ONION PANCAKES

½ tablespoon sunflower oil

3 bacon rashers/slices, cut into short strips

½ onion, finely chopped

100 g/3½ oz. button mushrooms, halved

225 g/1¾ cups plain/all-purpose flour

1 tablespoon baking powder

½ teaspoon salt

2 eggs

200 ml/generous ¾ cup whole milk

1 tablespoon freshly chopped parsley

1 tablespoon freshly chopped chives

25 g/2 tablespoons butter, melted

maple syrup, to serve (optional)

MAKES 16

Starting your weekend with a proper breakfast or a late brunch always feels like a treat. These small, fluffy pancakes – flavoured with mushrooms, bacon and onion – make a great savoury all-in-one breakfast dish to enjoy. Make a tall stack of them and share with friends.

Heat the sunflower oil in a frying pan/skillet. Add the bacon and onion and fry for 2 minutes over a medium heat, stirring. Add the mushrooms and fry over a high heat until lightly browned. Set aside to cool.

Sift the flour, baking powder and salt into a large mixing bowl. Break the eggs into the centre of the flour and pour in the milk, folding the ingredients together quickly, without over-mixing, to form a thick batter. Gently fold in the mushroom mixture, parsley and chives. Stir in the melted butter.

Thoroughly heat a large, heavy-based frying pan/skillet. Dry-fry the mixture in batches, using a tablespoon of the batter to form each small pancake. Fry for 2–3 minutes over a low-medium heat, until the pancakes have set and begun to dry out around the edges. Using a spatula, gently turn them over and fry for a further 2 minutes until golden brown on both sides. Serve at once with maple syrup, if you like.

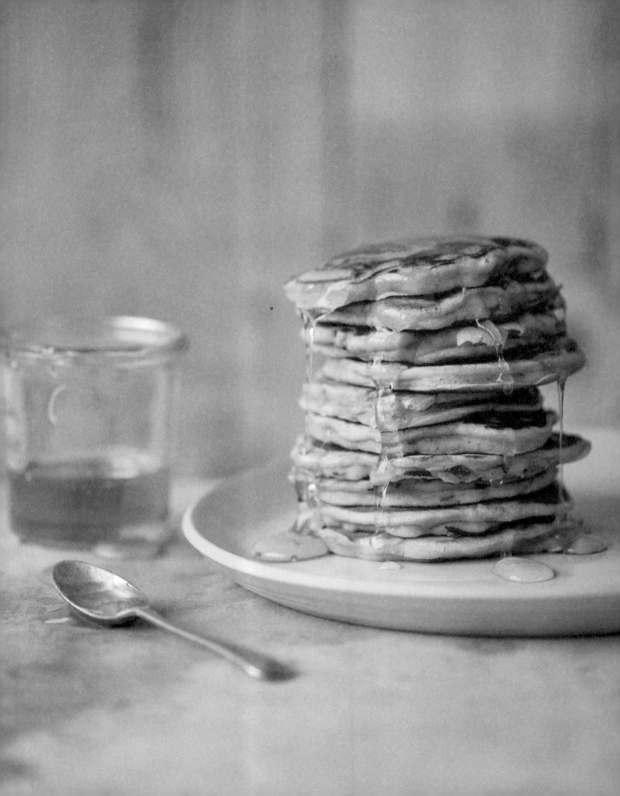

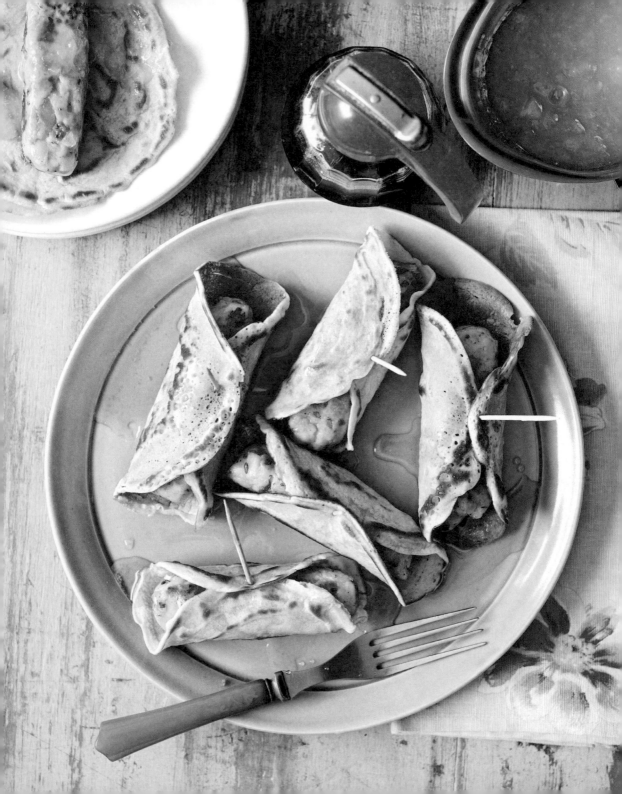

CHICKS IN A BLANKET

APPLESAUCE

4 green cooking apples, peeled, cored and chopped

60 g/scant ⅓ cup white sugar

½ teaspoon ground cinnamon

BREAKFAST SAUSAGES

15 g/1 tablespoon butter

1 sweet apple, peeled, cored and chopped

1 small white onion, finely chopped

1 teaspoon fennel seeds

700 g/1½ lbs. minced/ground chicken breast

1½ tablespoons freshly chopped sage

½ tablespoon light brown sugar

2 teaspoons olive oil

sea salt and freshly ground black pepper

PANCAKE BATTER

200 g/1½ cups plain/all-purpose flour

2 tablespoons white sugar

2 teaspoons baking powder

½ teaspoon bicarbonate of soda/baking soda

½ teaspoon salt

300–360 ml/1¼–1½ cups whole milk

2 eggs, beaten

30 g/2 tablespoons butter, melted

olive oil, for frying

maple syrup, to serve

SERVES 4

'Pigs in a blanket' is a slang term for pancakes wrapped around breakfast sausages. These 'chicks' are not made with pork sausage, but instead with chicken-apple breakfast sausages and served with a US-style applesauce.

To make the applesauce, combine the apples, sugar and cinnamon with 175 ml/¾ cup water in a saucepan over a medium heat. Cover and cook for 15–20 minutes or until the apples are soft. Allow to cool, then mash with a fork or potato masher. Set aside until ready to serve.

For the chicken-apple breakfast sausages, heat a small, non-stick frying pan/skillet over a medium heat. Add the butter and melt. Add the sweet apple and onion and season with a little salt and pepper and the fennel seeds. Gently cook the mixture for 5–7 minutes until softened. When cooked, remove from the heat and set aside.

Heat a large, non-stick frying pan/skillet over a medium-high heat. Place the chicken in a bowl and season well with salt and pepper, add the sage, sugar and olive oil. Add the apple, onion and fennel seed mixture and use your hands to mix well. Shape the mixture into 12 even sausages.

Fry the sausages in the frying pan/skillet for 3–4 minutes, then flip and cook for another 2–4 minutes, until cooked through. Remove from the pan and set aside, covered with foil, to keep warm.

To make the pancakes, in a bowl, mix together all the dry ingredients and make a well in the centre. Start with 300 ml/1¼ cups milk, adding up to another 60 ml/¼ cup if necessary, as you mix it with the flour. Add the beaten eggs and melted butter, combining with a whisk until well-mixed.

Heat a frying pan/skillet and add a little oil. When hot, pour in a ladleful of pancake mix at a time. When the pancake starts to bubble on top and is turning golden brown on the underside, turn it and continue cooking until both sides are golden brown. Repeat the cooking process with the remaining batter until you have 12 pancakes.

Keep the cooked pancakes covered with a clean kitchen cloth, to keep them warm while you finish cooking the rest. Once all the pancakes are cooked, wrap them around the sausages to form a roll with the sausages in the middle. Serve with maple syrup and the homemade applesauce.

HUEVOS RANCHEROS WAFFLES

WAFFLE BATTER

160 g/scant 1¼ cups self-raising/rising flour, sifted

100 g/1 cup fine polenta/cornmeal

1 teaspoon bicarbonate of soda/baking soda

1 tablespoon caster/granulated sugar

3 eggs, separated

375 ml/1⅔ cups whole milk

60 g/ ¼ cup butter, melted, plus extra for greasing

1 tablespoon olive or vegetable oil

8 eggs

70 g/scant 1 cup Cheddar cheese, grated

sour/soured cream, to serve

sea salt and freshly ground black pepper

SALSA

4 large tomatoes, halved

2 ripe avocados

freshly squeezed juice of 2 limes

2 heaped tablespoons freshly chopped coriander/cilantro

½ teaspoon hot paprika, plus extra for sprinkling

electric or stove-top waffle iron

SERVES 4

Huevos Rancheros or 'ranch eggs' are a traditional Mexican breakfast of spicy tomatoes with eggs served on corn tortillas. This version uses corn waffles in place of the tortillas. The tomato and avocado salsa provides a fresh twist on the classic dish in which the tomatoes are usually cooked. Wake up your senses with a kick of piquant paprika and the delicate fragrance of coriander/cilantro.

To make the waffle batter, put the flour, polenta/cornmeal, bicarbonate of soda/baking soda, sugar, the 3 egg yolks, the milk and melted butter in a large mixing bowl. Whisk until you have a smooth batter. Season with salt and pepper. In a separate mixing bowl, whisk the 3 egg whites to stiff peaks and then gently fold into the batter a third at a time.

Preheat the waffle iron and grease with a little butter.

Ladle some of the batter into the preheated waffle iron and cook for 2–3 minutes until golden brown. Keep the waffles warm while you cook the remaining batter and are ready to serve.

For the salsa, remove the seeds from the halved tomatoes using a teaspoon and discard. Cut the hollowed-out tomatoes into small pieces using a sharp knife. Prepare the avocados by removing the stones and skins and cutting the flesh into small pieces. Immediately mix the avocado with the lime juice and tomatoes so that it does not discolour. Add the coriander/cilantro, sprinkle over the paprika and stir in. Season with salt and pepper and set aside in the refrigerator until needed.

Heat the oil in a frying pan/skillet and fry the 8 eggs for 2–3 minutes until the whites of the eggs are cooked but the yolks are still soft.

Place the waffles on plates and top with a generous portion of the salsa. Place the fried eggs on top and sprinkle over the grated cheese. Top with a spoonful of sour cream and a pinch of paprika, and serve straight away.

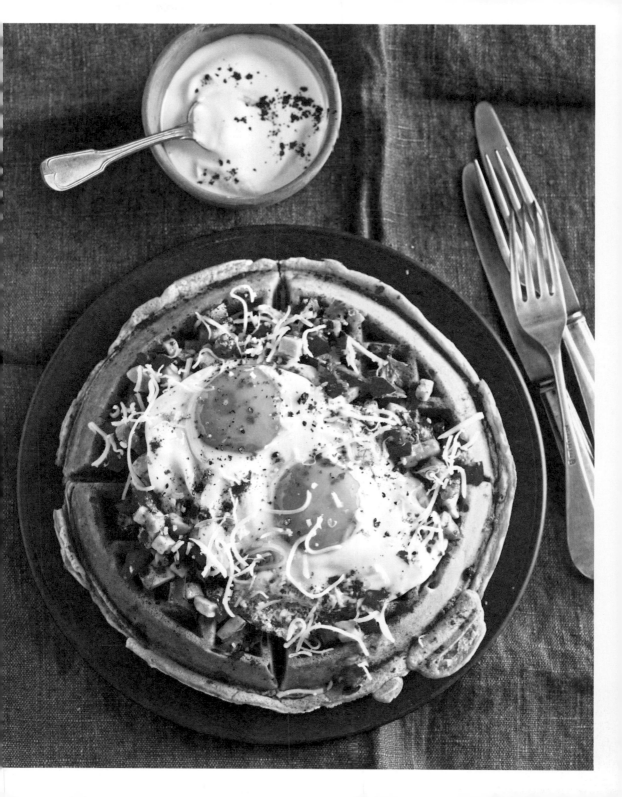

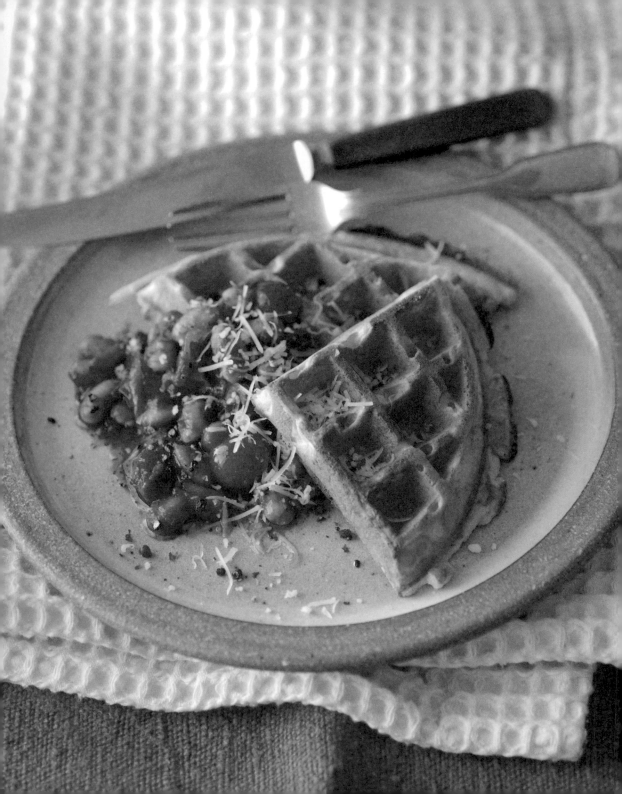

POTATO WAFFLES WITH BARBECUE BEANS

WAFFLE BATTER

2 baking potatoes

260 g/2 cups self-raising/rising flour, sifted

1 teaspoon baking powder

pinch of salt

3 eggs, separated

300 ml/1¼ cups milk

60 g/4 tablespoons butter, melted, plus extra for greasing

a handful of grated Cheddar or Emmental cheese, to serve

BARBECUE BEANS

1 tablespoon olive oil

1 medium onion, thinly sliced

1–2 garlic cloves, thinly sliced

400 g/2 cups canned chopped tomatoes

2 tablespoons Worcestershire sauce

2 tablespoons soy sauce

40 g/3¼ tablespoons dark brown sugar

480 g/3¾ cups cooked cannellini beans, drained and rinsed

sea salt and freshly ground black pepper

electric or stove-top waffle iron

baking sheet lined with baking parchment

SERVES 4

This recipe is breakfast-comfort-food-heaven with rich, saucy beans piled onto potato waffles and sprinkled liberally with grated cheese. The barbecue beans also make a great side dish for many other meals.

Preheat the oven to 200°C (400°F) Gas 6.

For the waffle batter, prick the potatoes with a fork and bake them in the preheated oven on the prepared baking sheet for 1 –1¼ hours (or in a microwave on full power for about 8 minutes per potato). Leave the potatoes to cool, then cut them open and remove the potato from the skins. Mash the flesh with a fork and set aside, discarding the skins.

To make the beans, heat the olive oil in a large saucepan set over a medium heat. Add the sliced onion and cook until it turns translucent. Add the garlic to the pan and cook for a few minutes longer until the onion and garlic are lightly golden brown. Add the tomatoes to the pan and season well with salt and pepper. Add the Worcestershire sauce, soy sauce and dark brown sugar and simmer until the sauce becomes thick and syrupy. Put the beans in the sauce and simmer for a further 20 minutes. Keep the pan on the heat but turn it down to low to keep the beans warm until you are ready to serve.

In a large mixing bowl, whisk together the cooled mashed potato, flour, baking powder, salt, egg yolks milk and melted butter until you have a smooth batter. In a separate bowl, whisk the egg whites to stiff peaks. Gently fold the whisked egg whites into the batter mixture using a spatula.

Preheat the waffle iron and grease with a little butter.

Ladle some of the batter into the preheated waffle iron and cook for 3–5 minutes until golden brown. Keep the waffles warm while you cook the remaining batter.

Serve the waffles topped with the hot barbecue beans and grated cheese.

BANANA PROTEIN PANCAKES
WITH CRISPY PARMA HAM

These little pancakes are both a delicious treat and a hit of protein to fuel you up for that gym session all in one! The delectable combination of sweet maple syrup with savoury Parma ham will set your taste buds alight!

PANCAKE BATTER
2 bananas, mashed

2 eggs

1 teaspoon vanilla extract (or the seeds from 1 vanilla pod/bean)

1 teaspoon ground cinnamon

2 tablespoons vanilla protein powder

1 tablespoon chia seeds

coconut oil (or coconut butter), for frying

TO SERVE
Parma ham/prosciutto

maple syrup

flaked/slivered almonds

MAKES 6

Mix all of the batter ingredients together well in a large mixing bowl and set aside for 10–15 minutes so the chia seeds can start to do their thing – they'll plump up and turn a little gelatinous when in contact with any moisture, and adding them here helps to thicken the batter.

Set a non-stick frying pan/skillet over a low-medium heat and add a little coconut oil or coconut butter. (Note that cooking these pancakes over a low-medium heat keeps them soft and springy, however, always make sure the pan is heated before adding the batter or the pancakes won't hold their shape and will become flat.)

You will need to cook the pancakes in batches of two or three. Pour even spoonfuls of the batter into the pan and when bubbles start to form on top, they should be ready to flip. Turn over using a spatula and cook the other side of each pancake.

Remove the pancakes from the pan as they are ready and keep them warm until you are ready to serve. In the same pan, fry the Parma ham prosciutto briefly over a high heat until crisp.

Serve the pancakes in stacks with a drizzle of maple syrup, a sprinkle of flaked/slivered almonds and topped with the crispy Parma ham/prosciutto. Enjoy.

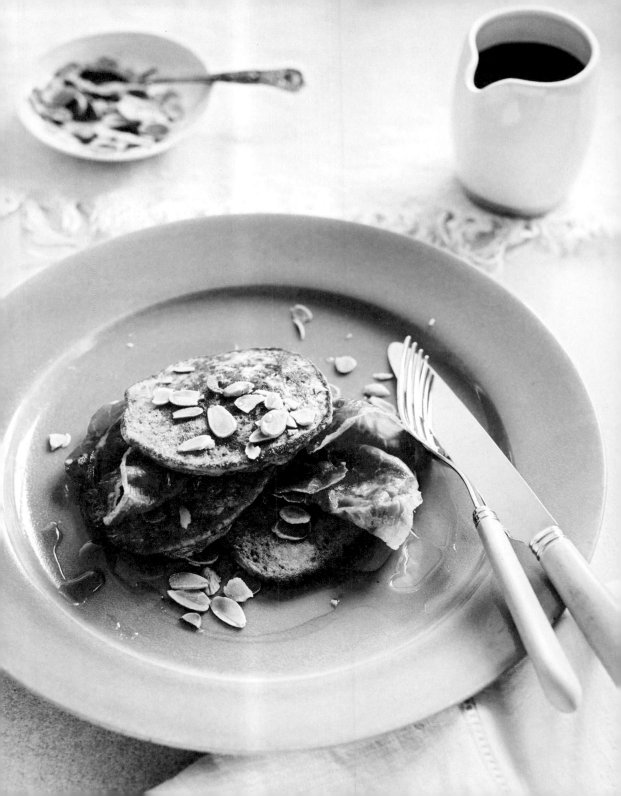

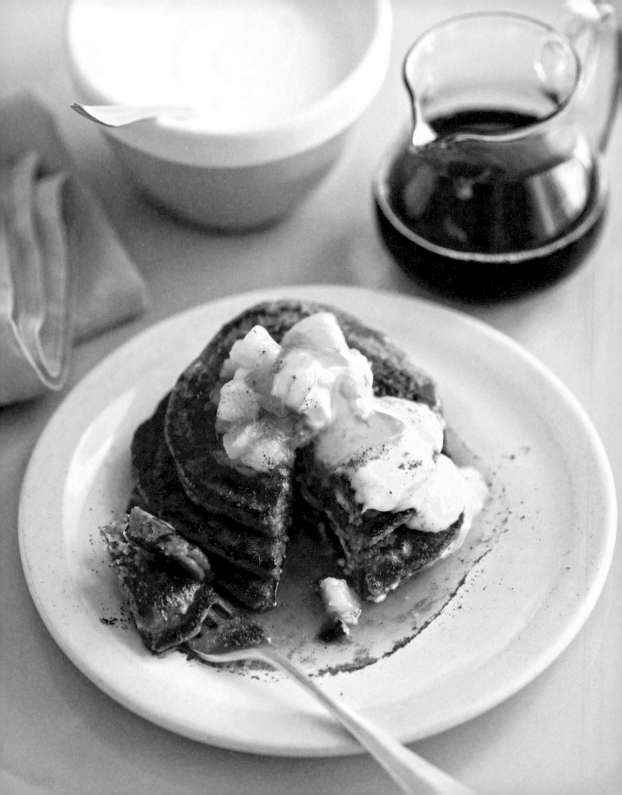

SWEET POTATO PANCAKES
WITH CINNAMON & VANILLA

If you are keen to get more fruit and vegetables into your diet, you might not have considered that pancakes can be one of your five-a-day. The sweet potato makes these pancakes naturally sweet and beautifully moist in texture, and they are a perfect flavour match with cinnamon and vanilla.

300 g/10½ oz. sweet potato, peeled and chopped

125 g/1 cup minus 1 tablespoon plain/all-purpose flour

1 teaspoon baking powder

1 teaspoon ground cinnamon

3–4 tablespoons caster/granulated sugar

1 tablespoon vanilla extract

125 ml/½ cup whole milk

1 egg, beaten

15 g/1 tablespoon butter, melted and slightly cooled

vegetable or groundnut (peanut) oil, for frying

yogurt, stewed apples and maple syrup, to serve

SERVES 4–6

Bring a pan of water to the boil and steam the sweet potatoes until tender, then drain and leave to cool. Meanwhile, sift the flour, baking powder and cinnamon into a large mixing bowl. Stir in the sugar. Add the vanilla extract to the milk and egg, along with the melted butter. Gradually add the wet ingredients to the dry, combining it all together with a fork. The batter can be made up to 24 hours in advance and stored in the refrigerator in a bowl, covered, if you like.

Before cooking, mash the sweet potatoes, then stir them through the batter until well combined. Melt a little oil in a non-stick frying pan/skillet over a fairly high heat. Once hot, carefully add heaped tablespoons of the batter. Gently fry the pancakes in batches until golden brown on both sides, turning them with a spatula. Remove the pancakes from the pan as they are ready and keep them warm until you are ready to serve.

Serve the pancakes in stacks with yogurt, stewed apples and maple syrup for a hearty breakfast.

GRANOLA PANCAKES
WITH SALTED HONEY SAUCE

PANCAKE BATTER

160 g/scant 1¼ cups self-raising/rising flour, sifted

1 teaspoon baking powder

1 egg, separated

1 tablespoon orange blossom honey

pinch of salt

250 ml/1 cup plus 1 tablespoon whole milk

3 tablespoons melted butter, plus extra for frying

120–150 g/1½ cups granola

SALTED HONEY SAUCE

60 g/4 tablespoons butter

3½ tablespoons runny honey

½ teaspoon salt

120 ml/½ cup double/heavy cream

MAKES 6

Granola gives an interesting crunchy, oaty top to these pancakes. They are served with a delicious, buttery, honey sauce. You can also add raisins, sultanas, dried berries and cherries to the batter for an extra fruity tang.

To make the pancake batter, put the flour, baking powder, egg yolk, honey, salt and milk in a large mixing bowl and whisk together. Add the melted butter and whisk again. The batter should have a smooth, dropping consistency.

In a separate bowl, whisk the egg white to stiff peaks. Gently fold the whisked egg white into the batter mixture using a spatula. Cover and put in the refrigerator to rest for 30 minutes.

To make the sauce, heat the butter and honey in a small saucepan until the butter has melted. Add the salt and whisk in the cream over the heat. Keep the pan on the heat, but turn it down to low to keep the sauce warm until you are ready to serve.

When you are ready to serve, remove your batter mixture from the refrigerator and stir once. Put a little butter in a large frying pan/skillet set over a medium heat. Allow the butter to melt and coat the base of the pan, then ladle the batter into the pan and sprinkle a little granola on top of the pancake. Cook until the underside of the pancake is golden brown and a few bubbles start to appear on the top – this will take about 2–3 minutes. Turn the pancake over using a spatula and cook on the other side until golden brown. Keep the pancake warm while you cook the remaining batter, adding more butter to the pan, if necessary.

Serve the pancakes with the warm honey sauce poured over the top.

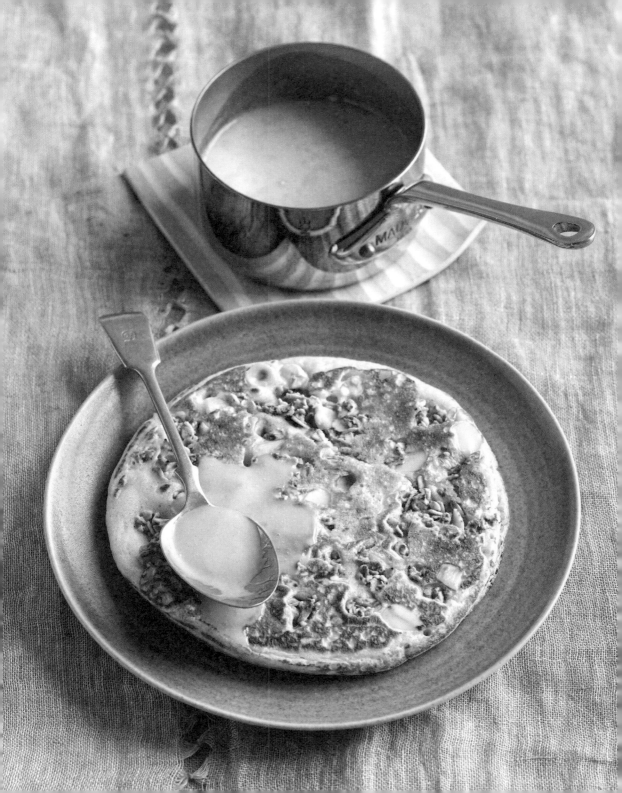

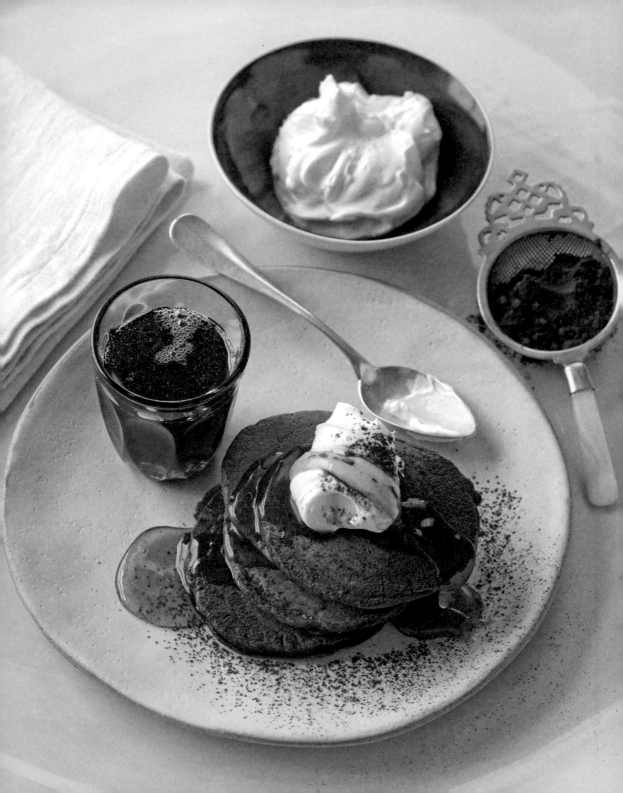

WAKE-ME-UP COFFEE PANCAKES

These are the perfect breakfast pancakes, with a real caffeine kick to wake you up in the morning. The coffee syrup is made with cocoa nibs which are fermented, dried, roasted cocoa pods. Cocoa nibs are both delicious and good for you as they don't contain sugar but still have an amazing chocolate taste. They are available from health food stores and some supermarkets, or online.

PANCAKE BATTER

160 g/scant 1¼ cups self-raising/rising flour, sifted

1 teaspoon baking powder

1 egg, separated

1 tablespoon caster/granulated sugar

pinch of salt

250 ml/1 cup plus 1 tablespoon iced milk coffee

3 tablespoons melted butter, plus extra for frying

150 g/1 cup mascarpone cheese

150 ml/²⁄₃ cup crème fraîche

icing/confectioners' sugar, to taste (optional)

cocoa powder, to dust

COFFEE SYRUP

100 ml/⅓ cup plus 1 tablespoon espresso coffee

60 ml/¼ cup coffee liqueur

100 g/½ cup caster/granulated sugar

1 teaspoon cocoa nibs or coffee beans

MAKES 12

Begin by making the coffee syrup. Put all of the syrup ingredients in a saucepan and simmer over a gentle heat for about 5 minutes until thick and gloopy. Set aside to allow the flavours to infuse and the syrup to cool.

To make the pancake batter, put the flour, baking powder, egg yolk, caster/granulated sugar, salt and iced coffee in a large mixing bowl and whisk together. Add the melted butter and whisk again. The batter should have a smooth, dropping consistency.

In a separate bowl, whisk the egg white to stiff peaks. Gently fold the whisked egg white into the batter mixture using a spatula. Cover and put in the refrigerator to rest for 30 minutes.

When you are ready to serve, remove your batter mixture from the refrigerator and stir once. Put a little butter in a large frying pan/skillet set over a medium heat. Allow the butter to melt and coat the base of the pan, then ladle small amounts of the batter into the pan, leaving a little space between each. Cook until the batter is just set, then turn over and cook for a further 2–3 minutes. Once cooked, keep the pancakes warm while you cook the remaining batter, adding a little butter to the pan each time, if required.

When you are ready to serve, place the mascarpone cheese and crème fraîche in a bowl, adding a little icing/confectioners' sugar to sweeten if you wish, and whisk together well.

Serve the pancakes in a stack with a dollop of the mascarpone cream on top and a drizzle of the syrup. Dust with a little cocoa powder and enjoy!

OATMEAL PANCAKES WITH BERRY COMPOTE

PANCAKE BATTER

370–400 ml/1¾ cups whole milk

200 g/1½ cups self-raising/ rising flour, sifted

2 teaspoons baking powder

1 egg

pinch of salt

1 tablespoon caster/granulated sugar

3 tablespoons melted butter, plus extra for frying

crème fraîche, to serve (optional)

BERRY COMPOTE

500 g/4 cups summer berries (raspberries, blueberries, strawberries and blackberries in any combination of your choosing), stalks removed

100 g/½ cup caster/granulated sugar

1 teaspoon vanilla extract

freshly squeezed juice of 1 lemon

TOASTED OATS

60 g/½ cup oatmeal

50 g/¼ cup caster/ granulated sugar

MAKES 10

In these substantial pancakes, oatmeal is soaked in milk and mixed into the batter. Served with a berry compote and crème fraîche, they are the perfect pancakes to make for a summer breakfast, when fresh berries are abundant.

Begin by preparing the compote. Put the berries in a saucepan set over a medium heat with 250 ml/1 cup plus 1 tablespoon water, the sugar, vanilla and lemon juice. Simmer until the sugar has dissolved and the fruit is just starting to soften but still holds its shape. This will take about 5 minutes. Set aside to cool, then store in the refrigerator until you are ready to serve.

To make the toasted oats, place the oats and sugar in a dry frying pan/ skillet over a medium heat and toast for a few minutes until the sugar starts to caramelize the oats. Remove from the heat and set aside to cool.

Soak half of the toasted oats in 250 ml/1 cup plus 1 tablespoon of the milk for about 30 minutes, until plump. Reserve the rest of the oats.

To make the pancake batter, put the flour, baking powder, egg, salt, sugar and milk-soaked oats in a large mixing bowl and whisk together. Add the melted butter and whisk again. Gradually add the remaining milk until you have a smooth, pourable batter. Be careful not to make the batter too thin when adding the remaining milk – you may not need it all. Cover and put in the refrigerator to rest for 30 minutes.

When you are ready to serve, remove your batter mixture from the refrigerator and stir. Put a little butter in a large frying pan/skillet over a medium heat. Allow the butter to melt and coat the base of the pan, then ladle small amounts of the batter into the pan. Sprinkle some of the reserved toasted oats over the top of the pancakes and cook until the underside of each is golden brown and a few bubbles start to appear on the top – this will take about 2–3 minutes. Turn the pancakes over using a spatula and cook on the other side until golden brown. Keep the pancakes warm while you cook the remaining batter in the same way.

Serve the pancakes with the berry compote and crème fraîche, if using.

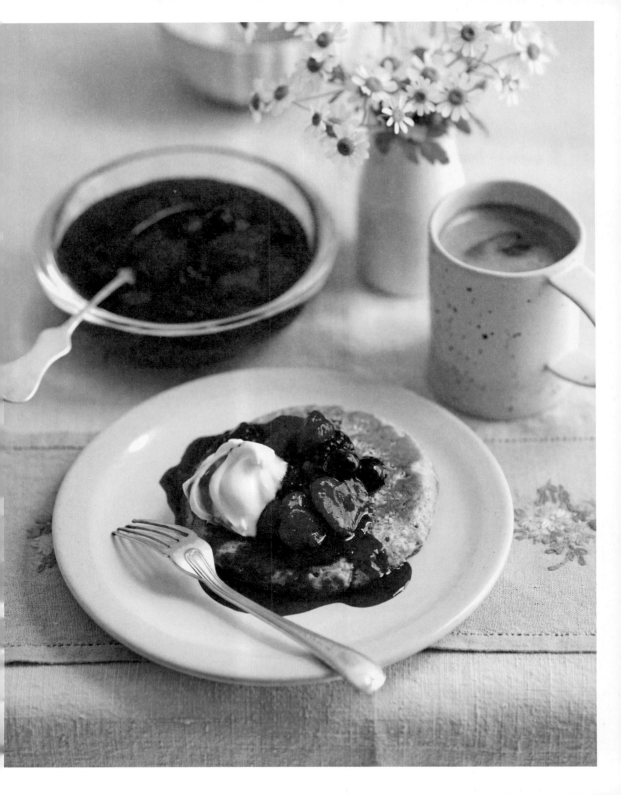

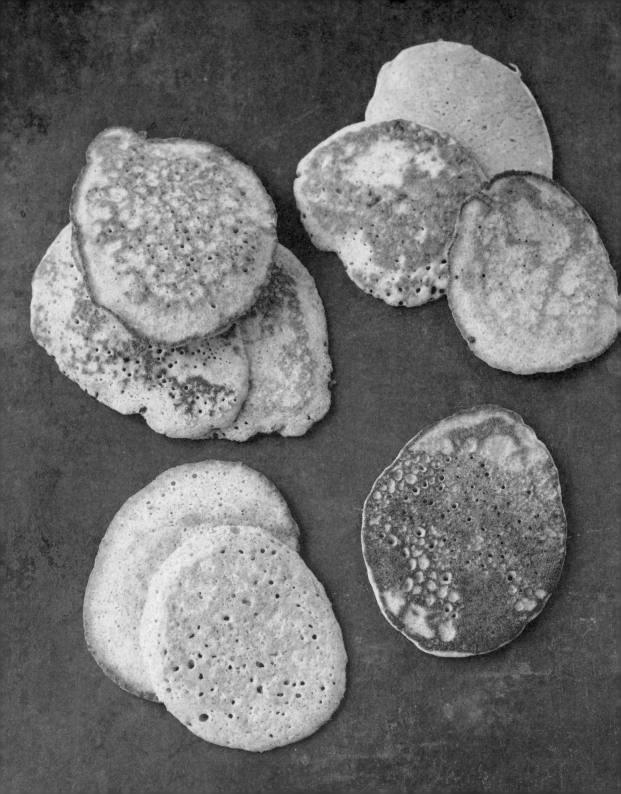

FEELING
FRUITY

DAIRY-FREE COCONUT PANCAKES
WITH LIME SYRUP & MANGO

These pancakes are completely dairy-free and egg-free. This makes them a bit more dense, but as they are served drenched in a lime and honey syrup, this is soon taken care of. Try to find the ripest, most perfumed mango you can to make this dish exquisite.

PANCAKE BATTER

150 g/1 cup plus 2 tablespoons plain/all-purpose flour

1 tablespoon baking powder

¼ teaspoon salt

2 tablespoons demerara/turbinado sugar

3 tablespoons desiccated/dried shredded coconut

200 ml/generous ¾ cup coconut milk

2 tablespoons sunflower oil, plus extra for frying

1 mango, peeled, destoned and sliced

LIME SYRUP

freshly squeezed juice of 3 limes

grated zest of 1 lime

100 g/6 tablespoons runny honey

6 cardamom pods, crushed

SERVES 4

To make the lime syrup, put the lime juice and zest, honey and cardamom pods in a small saucepan and bring to the boil. Boil for 5 minutes, then remove from the heat and set aside.

Meanwhile, for the pancake batter, sift the flour, baking powder and salt into a large mixing bowl and stir in the sugar and desiccated/dried shredded coconut. Put the coconut milk, 75 ml/⅓ cup water and the oil into a jug/pitcher and beat to combine. Mix the wet ingredients with the dry ingredients until no lumps of flour remain.

Heat a frying pan/skillet over a medium heat. Grease the pan with a paper towel dipped in oil. Drop 2–3 tablespoons of batter into the pan. Cook the pancakes for 1–2 minutes on each side until golden and cooked through. Remove the pancakes from the pan as they are ready and keep them warm while you cook the remaining batter in the same way.

Serve the pancakes with slices of fresh mango and the lime syrup.

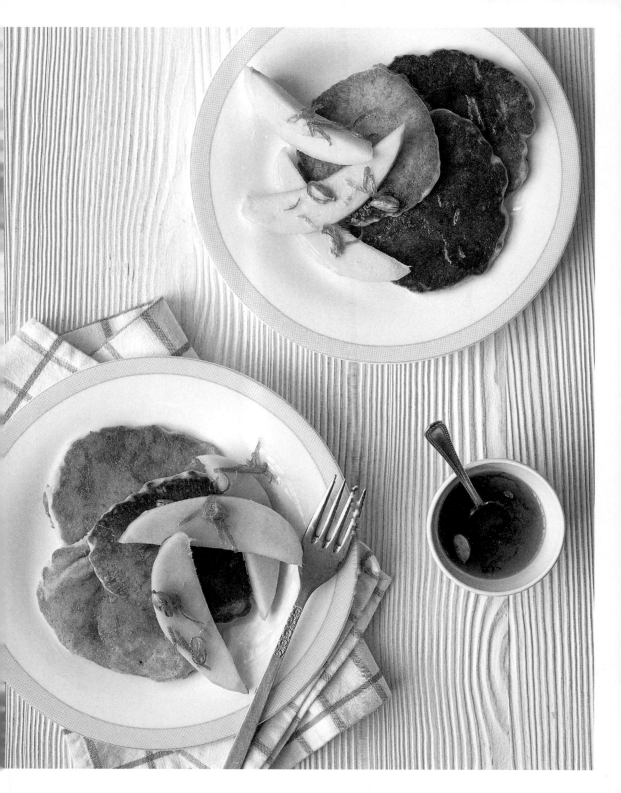

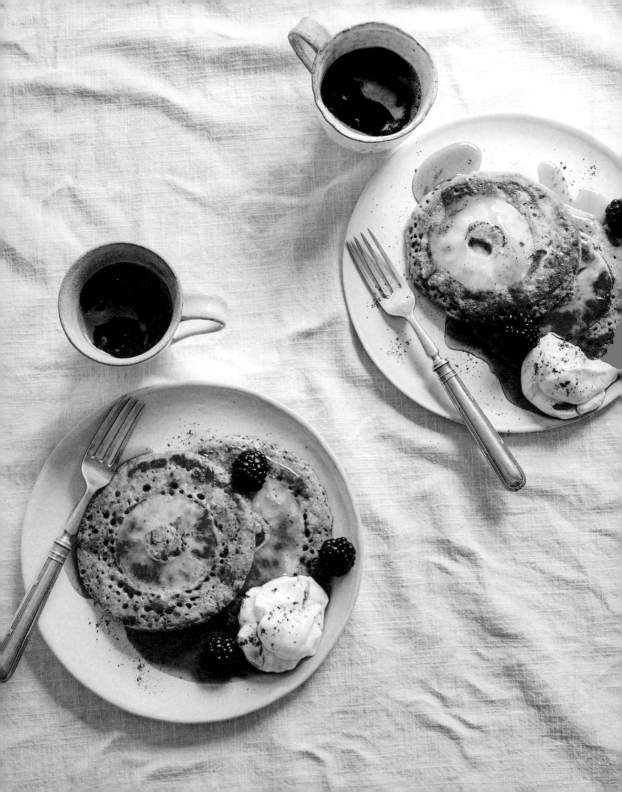

GLUTEN-FREE APPLE PANCAKES

These are quick to make and will be enjoyed by everyone, not just your gluten-free guests. The combination of the nuttiness of the buckwheat, the tartness of the apple and the mellow sweetness of maple syrup is a winner.

150 g/1 cup plus 2 tablespoons gluten-free plain/all-purpose flour

100 g/³⁄₄ cup buckwheat flour

1 tablespoon caster/granulated sugar

1 teaspoon gluten-free baking powder

pinch of salt

1 egg

220 ml/scant 1 cup whole milk

½ teaspoon vanilla extract

butter, for frying

1 Granny Smith apple, cored, peeled and sliced into rings

maple syrup, yogurt, vanilla powder and blackberries, to serve

SERVES 4

Put the flours, sugar, baking powder and salt in a large mixing bowl and make a well in the centre. Crack the egg into the middle and pour in a quarter of the milk. Use a whisk to combine the mixture thoroughly. Once you have a paste, mix in another quarter of the milk and, when all the lumps are gone, mix in the remaining milk and the vanilla extract. Leave to rest for 20 minutes. Stir again before cooking.

Heat a small, non-stick frying pan/skillet and add a knob/pat of butter. When the butter starts to foam, ladle some pancake batter into the centre of the pan forming a circle, then place an apple ring in the centre.

Cook for a few minutes until golden brown on the bottom and bubbles are bursting on the surface of the pancake, then turn over and cook until golden on the other side. Keep the pancakes warm while you cook the remaining batter in the same way, stirring the mixture between pancakes and adding more butter for frying, as necessary.

Serve with maple syrup, yogurt, vanilla powder and blackberries.

BUTTERMILK BLUEBERRY PANCAKES
WITH BLUEBERRY LIME SAUCE

Blueberries have a wonderful, explosive taste when fresh and in season, although they are available year-round in supermarkets and online. The lime juice in the sauce gives these pancakes an extra zing, although you might not need this if you have a batch of really tasty, fresh blueberries.

PANCAKE BATTER

160 g/scant 1¼ cups self-raising/rising flour, sifted

1 teaspoon baking powder

1 egg, separated

60 g/scant ⅓ cup minus 1 teaspoon caster/granulated sugar

pinch of salt

200 ml/generous ¾ cup whole milk

80 ml/5 tablespoons buttermilk

3 tablespoons melted butter, plus extra for frying

100 g/¾ cup fresh blueberries

BLUEBERRY LIME SAUCE

300 g/2¼ cups fresh blueberries

freshly squeezed juice of 3 limes

100 g/½ cup caster/granulated sugar

300 ml/1¼ cups double/heavy cream, whipped to soft peaks, to serve

MAKES 12

Begin by making the sauce. Place the blueberries, lime juice and caster/granulated sugar in a saucepan with 90 ml/6 tablespoons water, then simmer over a gentle heat for about 5–10 minutes until the fruit is soft and the sauce is thick and syrupy.

To make the pancake batter, put the flour, baking powder, egg yolk, caster/granulated sugar, salt, milk and buttermilk in a large mixing bowl and whisk together. Add the melted butter and whisk again. The batter should have a smooth, dropping consistency.

In a separate bowl, whisk the egg white to stiff peaks. Gently fold the whisked egg white into the batter mixture using a spatula. Cover and put in the refrigerator to rest for 30 minutes.

When you are ready to serve, remove your batter mixture from the refrigerator and stir once. Put a little butter in a large frying pan/skillet set over a medium heat. Allow the butter to melt and coat the base of the pan, then ladle small amounts of the batter into the pan, leaving a little space between each. Sprinkle a few blueberries over the top of the pancakes and cook until the underside of each pancake is golden brown and a few bubbles start to appear on the top – this will take about 2–3 minutes. Turn the pancakes over using a spatula and cook on the other side until golden brown. Keep the pancakes warm while you cook the remaining batter in the same way, adding a little more butter to the pan each time, if required, and sprinkling each pancake with blueberries.

Serve the pancakes in a stack, drizzled with the blueberry lime sauce and topped with a dollop of whipped cream.

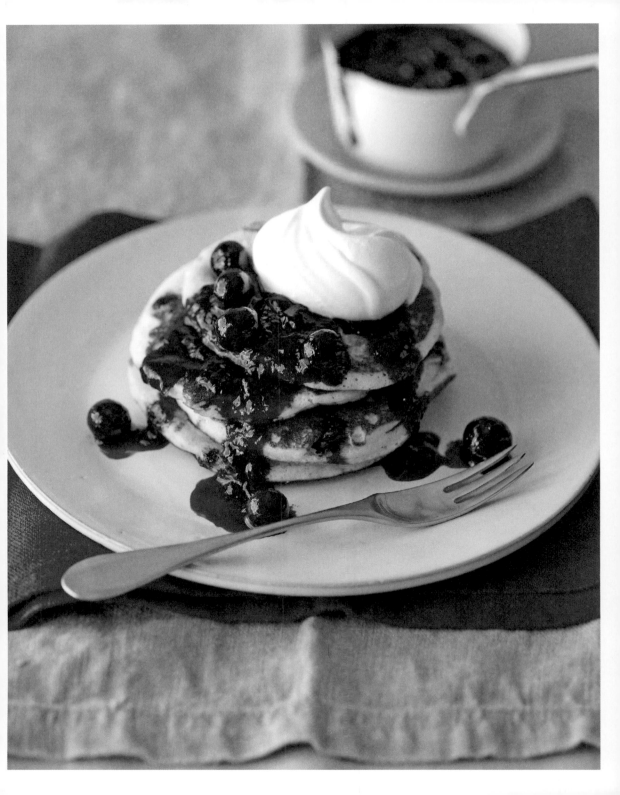

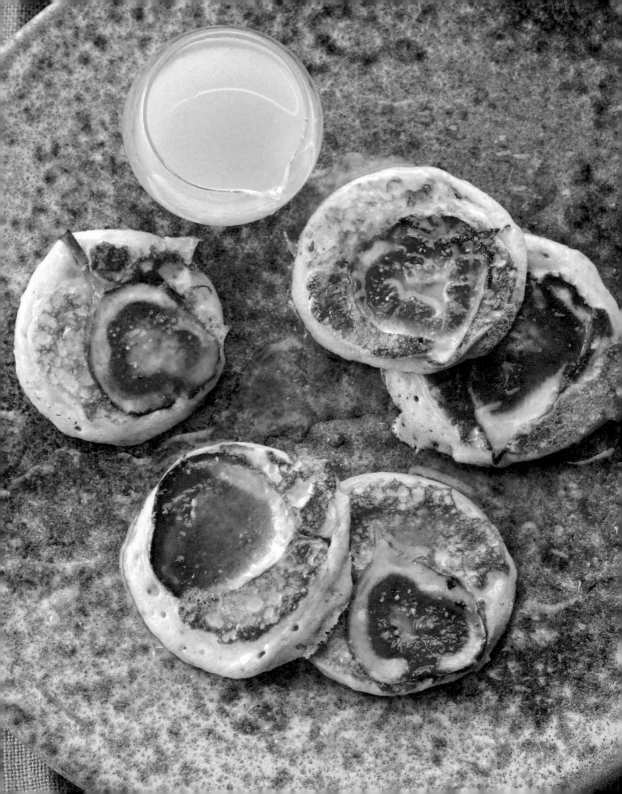

FIG & RICOTTA PANCAKES
WITH ORANGE SYRUP

The vibrant pink and green colours of the fresh figs nestled in the centre of these pancakes is reminiscent of summer, especially when served with sunny orange syrup. The ricotta makes them quite rich, so it is best to make them small and dainty enough to top with just one fig slice each.

PANCAKE BATTER

160 g/scant 1¼ cups self-raising/rising flour, sifted

1 teaspoon baking powder

2 eggs, separated

grated zest of 2 oranges

50 g/¼ cup caster/granulated sugar

pinch of salt

250 ml/1 cup plus 1 tablespoon whole milk

125 g/½ cup ricotta cheese

3 tablespoons melted butter, plus extra for frying

4–5 ripe figs, thinly sliced

sugar nibs/pearl sugar or caster/granulated sugar, for sprinkling

ORANGE SYRUP

freshly squeezed juice of 4 oranges

100 g/½ cup caster/granulated sugar

50 g/3½ tablespoons butter

MAKES 18

Begin by preparing the syrup. Put the orange juice, sugar and butter in a saucepan over a medium heat and simmer until the sugar is melted. Keep the pan on the heat, but turn it down to low to keep the syrup warm until you are ready to serve.

To make the pancake batter, put the flour, baking powder, egg yolks, orange zest, caster/granulated sugar, salt, milk and ricotta cheese in a large mixing bowl and whisk together. Add in the melted butter and whisk again. The batter should have a smooth, dropping consistency.

In a separate bowl, whisk the egg whites to stiff peaks. Gently fold the whisked egg whites into the batter mixture using a spatula. Cover and put in the refrigerator to rest for 30 minutes.

When you are ready to serve, remove your batter mixture from the refrigerator and stir once. Put a little butter in a large frying pan/skillet set over a medium heat. Allow the butter to melt and coat the base of the pan, then ladle small spoonfuls of batter into the pan, leaving a little space between each. Place a slice of fig on top of each pancake and sprinkle with sugar nibs/pearl sugar or caster/granulated sugar. Cook until the underside of each pancake is golden brown and a few bubbles start to appear on the top – this will take about 1–2 minutes. Turn the pancakes over using a spatula and cook on the other side until the sugar-topped figs have caramelized and the tops are golden brown. Keep the pancakes warm while you cook the remaining batter in the same way.

Serve the pancakes immediately with a drizzle of the orange syrup.

COCONUT & CHOCOLATE PANCAKES

With crunchy toasted, shredded coconut as well as coconut syrup, these pancakes are a coconut-lover's dream, and chocolate chips are a perfect partner too. If you cannot find long shredded soft coconut, you can use desiccated/dried shredded coconut instead.

PANCAKE BATTER

160 g/scant 1¼ cups self-raising/rising flour, sifted

1 teaspoon baking powder

1 egg, separated

1 teaspoon vanilla extract

60 g/⅓ cup minus 1 teaspoon caster/granulated sugar

pinch of salt

250 ml/1 cup plus 1 tablespoon whole milk

3 tablespoons melted butter, plus extra for frying

100 g/⅔ cup plain/bittersweet or milk/semi-sweet chocolate chips

150 g/2 cups long shredded soft coconut

COCONUT SYRUP

200 ml/generous ¾ cup coconut milk

75 g/⅓ cup plus 2 teaspoons caster/granulated sugar

MAKES 6

To make the pancake batter, put the flour, baking powder, egg yolk, vanilla, caster/granulated sugar, salt and milk in a large mixing bowl and whisk together. Add in the melted butter and whisk again. The batter should have a smooth, dropping consistency.

In a separate bowl, whisk the egg white to stiff peaks. Gently fold the whisked egg white, the chocolate chips and half of the shredded coconut into the batter mixture using a spatula. Cover and put in the refrigerator to rest for 30 minutes.

Toast the remaining coconut in a dry frying pan/skillet until lightly golden brown. Take care to watch it closely as it can burn easily.

For the sauce, put the coconut milk and sugar in a saucepan set over a medium heat and simmer for about 5 minutes until the mixture turns syrupy. Keep the pan on the heat, but turn it down to low to keep the sauce warm until you are ready to serve.

When you are ready to serve, remove your batter mixture from the refrigerator and stir gently. Put a little butter in a large frying pan/skillet set over a medium heat. Allow the butter to melt and coat the base of the pan, then ladle a little of the batter into the pan. Sprinkle a tablespoon of toasted coconut over the top of the pancake and cook until the underside is golden brown and a few bubbles start to appear on the top – this will take about 2–3 minutes. Turn the pancake over using a spatula and cook on the other side until golden brown. Keep the pancake warm while you cook the remaining batter in the same way, adding a little more butter to the pan each time, if required.

Serve the pancakes warm, sprinkled with the remaining toasted coconut and a drizzle of coconut sauce.

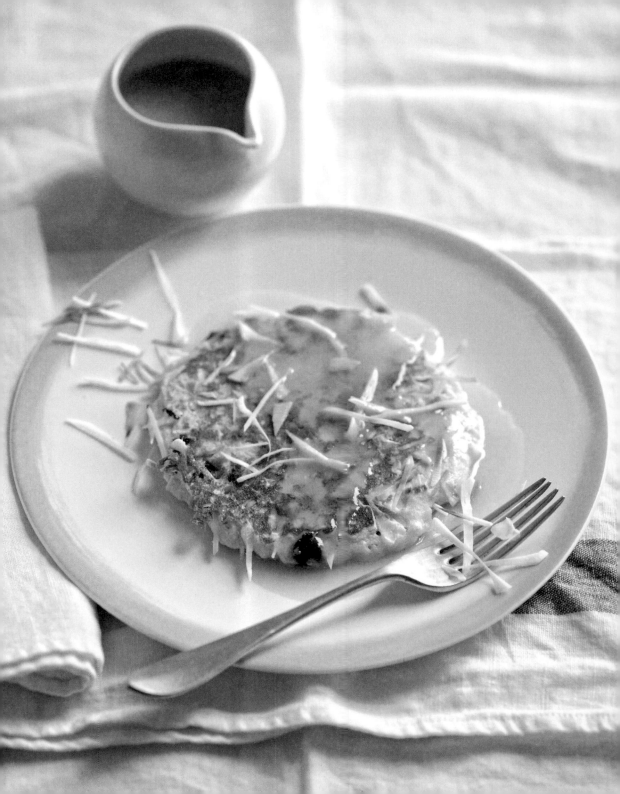

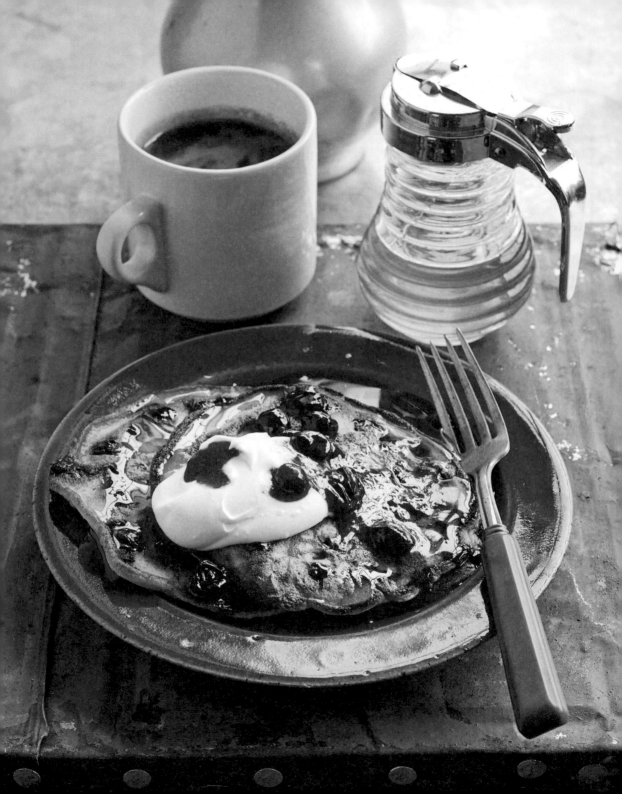

BLUEBERRY COTTON CANDY PANCAKES

Blueberry cotton candy pancakes mix a little bit of fairground nostalgia into breakfast, so this dish is perfect for a dreary Monday morning. The tartness of the blueberries balances out the sweet flavour of the cotton candy flavouring to make a fun breakfast, dessert or snack.

PANCAKE BATTER
200 g/1½ cups plain/
   all-purpose flour
1 tablespoon caster/granulated
   sugar
1 tablespoon brown sugar
1 teaspoon baking powder
½ teaspoon bicarbonate of
   soda/baking soda
½ teaspoon salt
2 eggs, at room temperature
250 ml/1 cup plus 1 tablespoon
   whole milk
235 g/1 cup sour/soured cream
   or plain/natural yogurt
115 g/1 stick butter, melted
6 drops cotton candy flavouring
½ teaspoon vanilla extract
225 g/1½ cups fresh blueberries,
   plus extra to serve
maple syrup, to serve

MAPLE WHIPPED CREAM
500 ml/2 cups plus 2
   tablespoons double/
   heavy cream
1½ tablespoons maple syrup

SERVES 4

Sift or whisk the dry ingredients (flour, sugars, baking powder, bicarbonate of soda/baking soda and salt) for the pancake batter together in a mixing bowl. In a separate bowl, lightly whisk the eggs. Add the milk and the sour/soured cream or yogurt, half the melted butter, the cotton candy flavouring and the vanilla, whisking to incorporate.

Make a well in the centre of the dry ingredients and pour the egg mixture into it. Whisk the ingredients together until combined, then fold the blueberries into the batter.

Heat a large frying pan/skillet over a medium heat and coat with some of the remaining melted butter. Pour a small ladleful of the batter into the centre of the pan. When bubbles begin to form and burst on the pancake's surface, after about 1 minute, and the outer edge looks done, flip it over and cook briefly for about 30 seconds on the other side. Remove the pancake from the pan as it is ready and keep warm until ready to serve. Repeat until the batter is used up, adding a little butter to the pan each time before adding the batter.

To make the maple whipped cream, add the cream and the maple syrup to a mixing bowl and whisk with a hand-held electric mixer until the whipped cream forms soft peaks.

Serve the pancakes with the maple whipped cream, extra maple syrup and fresh blueberries.

VENDOR-STYLE BANANA PANCAKES

This style of banana pancake is ubiquitous across the Indian subcontinent and South-east Asia as a trusted go-to snack. The authentic street-food style pancake is not made with egg, but a sweetened roti dough; you can use ready-made roti if you want to save time. Stuff with chocolate spread or peanut butter or serve with cream and golden/light corn syrup, as preferred.

270 g/2 cups plain/all-purpose flour

1–2 teaspoons sugar, to taste

½ teaspoon salt

150 ml/⅔ cup vegetable oil, plus extra to grease

2–3 ripe bananas, peeled and thickly sliced

chocolate spread (optional)

peanut butter (optional)

cream and golden/light corn syrup , to serve (optional)

MAKES 4

Put the flour in a bowl and add the sugar and salt. Mix together well, then add enough cold water to make a soft dough (about 150 ml/⅔ cup). Knead until soft, then add 1 tablespoon of the oil and knead for a good 10 minutes. Cover the dough with a damp kitchen cloth and leave to rest for at least 2 hours.

Grease the work surface with oil, then roll out the dough into well-oiled balls about the size of golf balls. Roll out each ball to make a flatbread about 12 cm/4½ inches in diameter. Leave to rest for 10 minutes.

Take each flatbread and, using your hands, stretch the dough as thinly as possible while continually smearing the dough with oil. It doesn't matter if the dough tears, but it's important to stretch it out thinly. Fold the dough back over itself in layers, to make a rough square about 10 cm/4 inches wide. Roll the dough out as thinly as possible to fit your largest frying pan/skillet.

Heat the frying pan/skillet over a medium heat and cook the pancake on one side (do not cook it too much at this stage, as it will make it difficult to fold the pancake), then turn it over and add some of the banana, chocolate spread or peanut butter, if using, into the centre, filling about half the pancake.

Fold in the sides of the pancake to form a thick rectangle, then cook gently on all sides until golden brown and the sweet dough is well cooked, adding more oil if necessary. Drain for 1–2 minutes on paper towels. Repeat with the remaining dough balls. Slice each pancake in half at an angle, then serve drizzled with cream and golden/light corn syrup for an extra sweet hit, if you like.

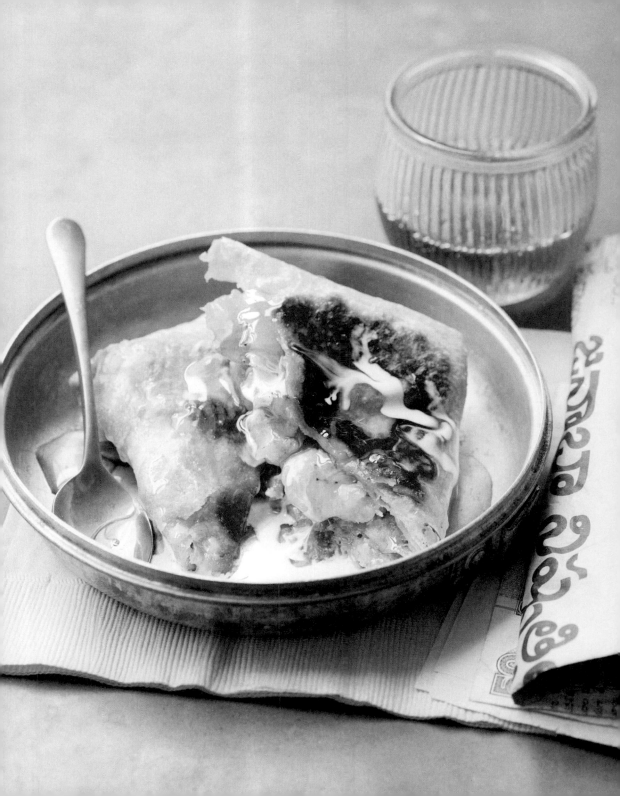

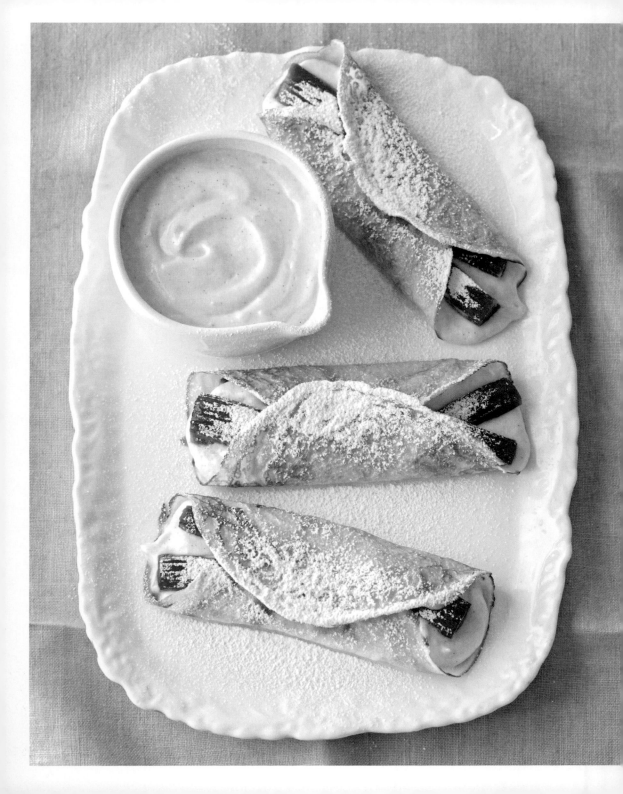

RHUBARB & CUSTARD CRÊPES

CRÊPE BATTER

140 g/1 cup plus 1 tablespoon plain/all-purpose flour, sifted

1 egg and 1 egg yolk

2 tablespoons melted butter, cooled, plus extra for frying

15 g/4 teaspoons caster/granulated sugar

pinch of salt

300 ml/1¼ cups whole milk

icing/confectioners' sugar, to dust

ROASTED RHUBARB

800 g/20 sticks pink rhubarb, ends trimmed

2 tablespoons caster/granulated sugar

CUSTARD

4 egg yolks

80 g/scant ½ cup caster/granulated sugar

2 tablespoons cornflour/cornstarch, sifted

1 vanilla pod/bean, halved and seeds removed

300 ml/1¼ cups double/heavy cream

250 ml/1 cup plus 1 tablespoon whole milk

ovenproof dish, greased

crêpe swizzle stick (optional)

MAKES 10

Tangy, pink rhubarb and creamy custard perfectly complement each other. This combination makes a great pancake filling with lashings of homemade custard to pour over. You can make both the rhubarb and custard in advance and cook the pancakes just before serving.

Begin by preparing the roasted rhubarb. Preheat the oven to 170°C (325°F) Gas 3. Put the rhubarb in the prepared ovenproof dish. Sprinkle with the sugar and pour over 120 ml/½ cup water. Bake in the preheated oven for 30–40 minutes until the rhubarb is soft but still holds its shape.

Meanwhile, for the crêpe batter, put the flour, egg and egg yolk, melted butter, caster/granulated sugar and salt in a large mixing bowl. Whisking all the time, gradually add the milk until you have a smooth and runny batter. Cover and put the batter in the refrigerator to rest for 30 minutes.

While the batter is resting, make the custard. Place the egg yolks, sugar and cornflour/cornstarch in a mixing bowl and whisk until very light and creamy. Set aside. Put the prepared vanilla pod/bean and seeds in a saucepan with the cream and milk over a high heat. Bring to the boil, then, whisking continuously, pour the hot milk over the egg mixture. Whisk well and then return to the pan. Stir over a gentle heat for a few minutes, until thickened. Remove the vanilla pod/bean and leave to cool.

Remove the batter from the refrigerator and stir gently. Put a little butter in a large frying pan/skillet set over a medium heat. Allow the butter to melt and coat the base of the pan, then ladle a small amount of the rested batter into the pan and spread it out thinly. You can do this either by tilting the pan, or, for best results, use a crêpe swizzle stick. Cook until the top of the crêpe is set, then turn over very carefully with a spatula and cook on the other side for a further 1–2 minutes until the crêpe is golden brown. Keep the crêpe warm while you cook the remaining batter in the same way, adding a little butter each time as needed.

Fill each crêpe with a little custard and two sticks of roasted rhubarb, then roll up. Dust with icing/confectioners' sugar and serve with the remaining custard on the side.

PEAR & GINGER WAFFLES

WAFFLE BATTER

260 g/2 cups self-raising/rising flour, sifted

1 teaspoon ground ginger

60 g/scant ⅓ cup caster/granulated sugar

pinch of salt

3 eggs, separated

375 ml/1⅔ cups whole milk

2 tablespoons ginger syrup

60 g/4 tablespoons butter, melted, plus extra for greasing

icing/confectioners' sugar, to dust

ginger or maple syrup, to drizzle

POACHED PEARS

4 ripe pears, peeled and cored, stalk intact

3 balls stem ginger preserved in syrup

80 ml/5 tablespoons ginger wine

2 tablespoons caster/granulated sugar

GINGER CREAM

2 balls stem ginger, finely chopped, plus 1 tablespoon of the preserving ginger syrup

300 ml/1¼ cups double/heavy cream

electric or stove-top waffle iron

MAKES 8

The piquant ginger spice runs throughout this recipe in its many forms – ground, stem, ginger syrup and ginger wine. If you love ginger, then this is the recipe for you. Although the poached pears are delicious, if you are short of time, you can substitute sliced, fresh pears instead.

Begin by preparing the pears. Put the pears in a saucepan with the stem ginger, ginger wine and sugar and then add water to the pan until the pears are covered. Set over a medium heat and simmer for 20–30 minutes until the pears are soft. Drain the pears, discarding the liquid and stem ginger, and set aside to cool. Once cool, cut each pear in half, cutting through the stalk so that each pear half still has part of the stalk at the top. Thinly slice each pear half but don't cut all the way through – you can then fan the pears out on top of the waffles. Set aside until ready to serve.

To make the ginger cream, put the ginger syrup and cream in a mixing bowl and whip to soft peaks. Fold the ginger pieces into the mixture and store in the refrigerator until you are ready to serve.

To make the waffle batter, put the flour, ginger, caster/granulated sugar, salt, egg yolks, milk, ginger syrup and melted butter in a large mixing bowl. Whisk until you have a smooth batter. In a separate mixing bowl, whisk the egg whites to stiff peaks and then gently fold into the batter, a third at a time.

Preheat the waffle iron and grease with a little butter.

Ladle a small amount of the batter into the preheated waffle iron and cook the waffles for 2–3 minutes until golden brown. Keep the waffles warm while you cook the remaining batter in the same way.

Serve the waffles immediately with a spoonful of the ginger cream and one poached pear half each. Dust with icing/confectioners' sugar and drizzle with a little ginger or maple syrup.

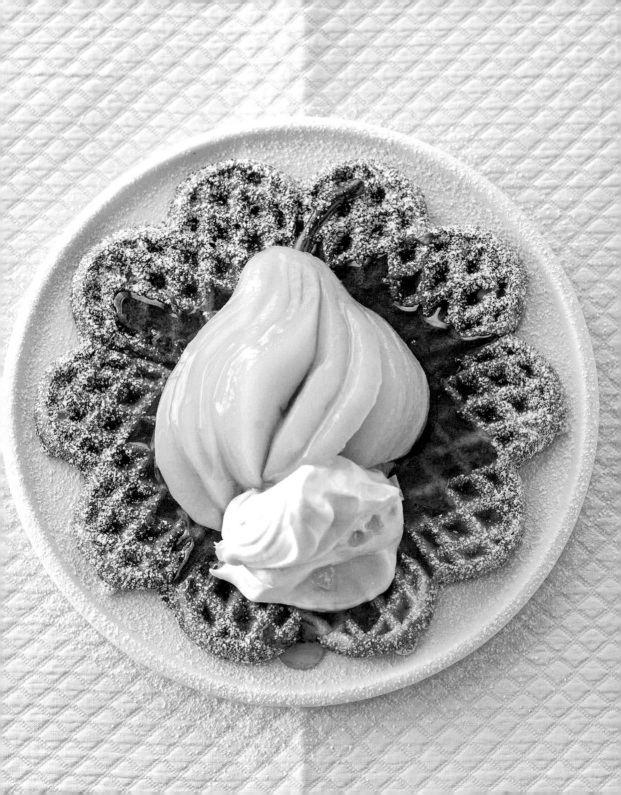

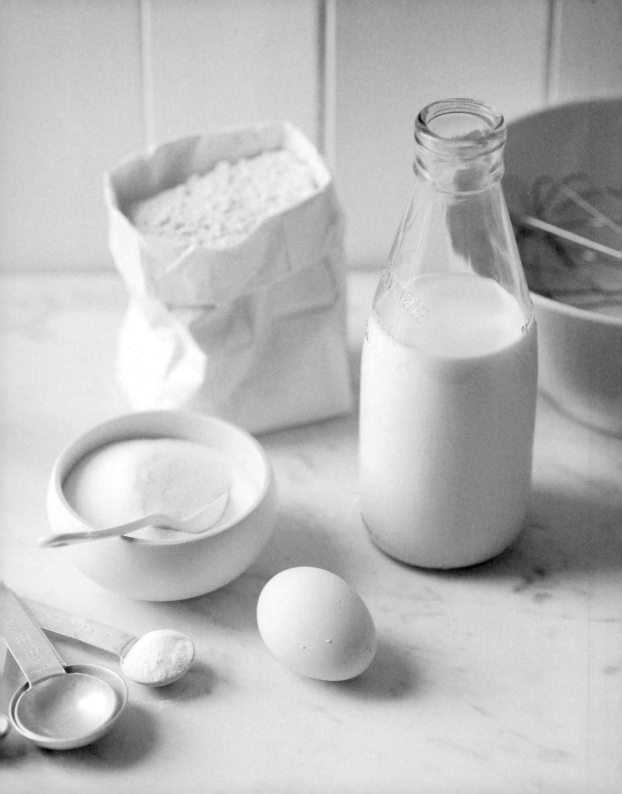

FLIPPING NUTRITIOUS

SEEDED BAKED PANCAKE
WITH BERRIES & COCOA SAUCE

PANCAKE BATTER

50 g/generous ⅓ cup
   plain/all-purpose flour

3 tablespoons coconut flour

1 teaspoon baking powder

pinch of salt

150 ml/⅔ cup milk

3 eggs, beaten

4 tablespoons runny honey

1 teaspoon vanilla extract

5 tablespoons mixed seeds,
   such as linseeds, chia seeds,
   sunflower seeds, poppy seeds

2 tablespoons coconut oil

COCOA SAUCE

4 tablespoons raw cocoa
   powder

2½ tablespoons runny honey

2½ tablespoons coconut oil,
   melted

TO SERVE

150 g/¾ cup Greek yogurt

50 g/1¾ oz. dried berries, such
   as goji, acai, cranberries etc.

100 g/3½ oz. mixed fresh
   berries such as blueberries,
   raspberries, redcurrants etc.

icing/confectioners' sugar

*22-cm/9-inch ovenproof
   frying pan/skillet*

SERVES 4

Based on the Dutch pancake that is baked in the oven, this is a super-easy and delicious way to make a pancake to serve straight from the pan. This one is packed full of nutritious seeds and served with berries and a healthyish cocoa sauce for a truly power-packed breakfast or dessert.

Preheat the oven to 200°C (400°F) Gas 6.

To make the pancakes, sift the plain/all-purpose flour, coconut flour, baking powder and salt into a mixing bowl. Combine the milk, eggs, honey and vanilla in a separate bowl and beat into the flours to make a smooth batter. Fold in the mixed seeds.

Heat the coconut oil in the ovenproof frying pan/skillet until melted. Pour in the pancake batter and transfer to the oven. Bake in the preheated oven for 15 minutes until the pancake is puffed up and golden.

Meanwhile, make the cocoa sauce. Place all the ingredients with 4 tablespoons water in a saucepan and heat gently, stirring, until smooth. Keep warm.

As soon as the pancake is cooked, remove it from the oven. Spoon the yogurt into the centre and top with the dried and fresh berries. Drizzle over the cocoa sauce and serve dusted with icing/confectioners' sugar.

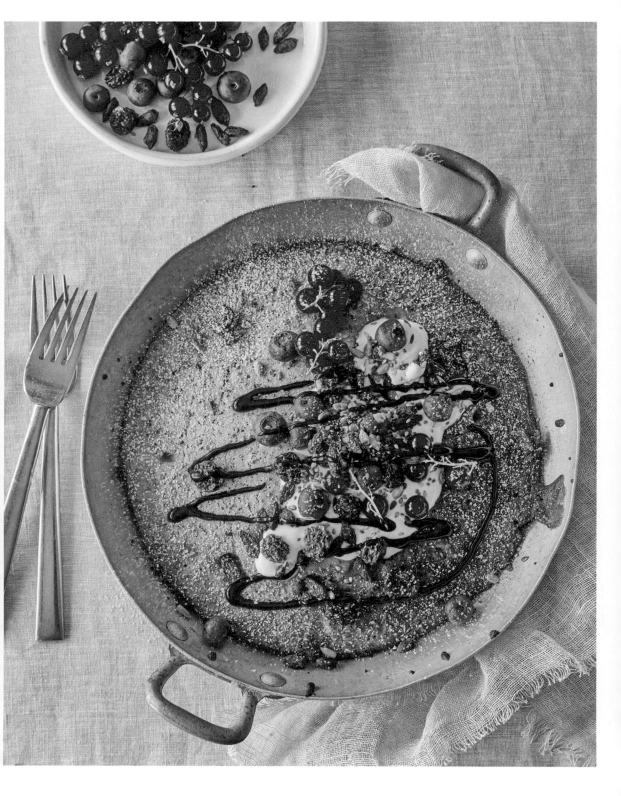

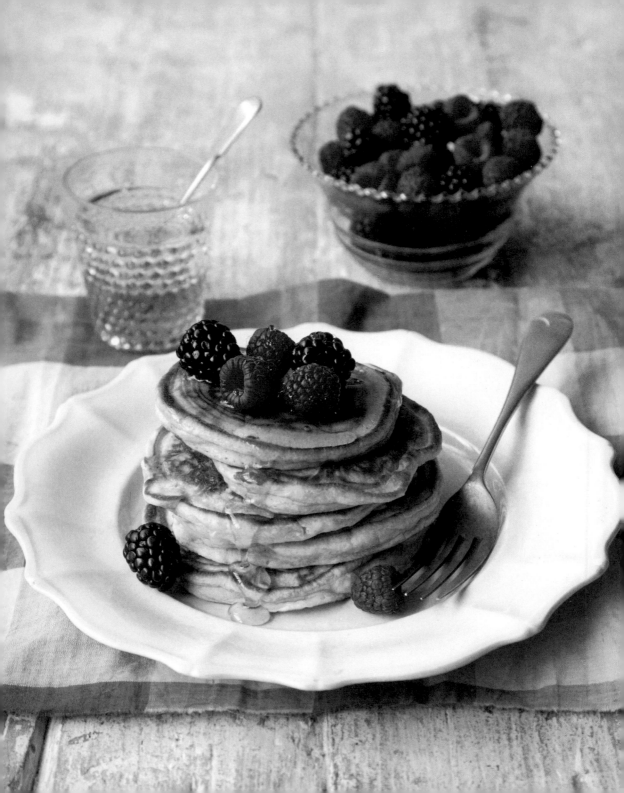

PROTEIN PANCAKES

Who doesn't love a pancake? With a healthifying makeover, you can have these any day of the week rather than saving them for an indulgent Sunday brunch. When you are wiped out at the end of the day, you can even whip these up for dinner and not feel the slightest bit guilty about it...

6 tablespoons plain/all-purpose flour

1 scoop of protein powder of choice

½ tablespoon xylitol or stevia, or other granulated sweetener

½ teaspoon baking powder

pinch of salt

1 small banana, peeled

1 tablespoon non-dairy milk of choice

1 teaspoon vanilla extract

½ teaspoon coconut oil

berries of choice and maple syrup, or dark/bittersweet chocolate chips, to serve

SERVES 1

In a bowl, combine the flour, protein powder, sweetener, baking powder and salt.

In a separate bowl, mash the banana until no lumps remain, then add the milk and vanilla extract.

Mix the wet ingredients into the bowl of dry ingredients until combined.

Melt the coconut oil in a frying pan/skillet over a medium heat so that it coats the bottom of the pan. Spoon a quarter of the pancake batter at a time into the pan, then flip the pancake over when you see it start to bubble. Cook until golden underneath. Remove the pancake from the pan and keep it warm while you make the remaining pancakes with the rest of the batter.

Serve with berries and a touch of maple syrup for a healthy option, or dark/bittersweet chocolate chips for a treat.

BUCKWHEAT PANCAKES
WITH PEARS IN CHAI SYRUP

PANCAKE BATTER

200 g/1½ cups buckwheat flour

50 g/¼ cup maple sugar or
    light brown sugar

2 teaspoons baking powder

pinch of kosher/rock salt

350 ml/1½ cups whole milk

1 teaspoon vanilla extract

2 tablespoons melted butter

1 egg

vegetable oil, for frying

PEARS IN CHAI SYRUP

2 black tea bags or 2
    tablespoons loose black tea

1 teaspoon cloves

½ teaspoon ground allspice

10 cardamom pods, bashed

1 teaspoon ground ginger

½ teaspoon ground cinnamon

4 star anise

½ teaspoon whole black
    peppercorns

300 g/1½ cups cane sugar

6 firm pears, cut into wedges
    and cores removed

SERVES 4

Buckwheat flour gives these pancakes a nutty taste. Topped with amazing syrupy pears infused with chai spices, it just doesn't get any better. A great brunch dish, but also sumptuous enough to serve as dessert with plenty of ice cream on the side.

Begin by making the pears in chai syrup. Place the tea, cloves, allspice, cardamom, ginger, cinnamon, star anise, peppercorns, sugar and 1.4 litres/6 cups water in a saucepan. Bring to the boil, then reduce the heat and simmer for 20 minutes, stirring occasionally. Remove the pan from the heat and set aside for 1 hour or overnight for a deeper flavour.

Strain the cooled chai through a fine mesh sieve/strainer and return to the pan. Bring to the boil, then reduce the heat to a simmer. Place the pears in the pan and gently cook for 15 minutes until tender. Keep the pears warm over a low heat while you make the pancakes. (Note: any leftover pears in syrup will keep in the refrigerator for up to 3 days).

For the pancake batter, place the flour, sugar, baking powder and salt in a bowl and mix together. In a separate bowl, whisk together the milk, vanilla, butter and egg. Pour the milk mixture into the flour mixture and whisk until just combined.

Heat a skillet/frying pan over a medium-high heat and drizzle with a little vegetable oil. Using a measuring cup or jug/pitcher, pour in 60 ml/ ¼-cup quantities of batter, two at a time, into the pan. When bubbles start appearing on the top of the pancakes, flip them over and press down gently on the tops with the back of the spatula. Cook for 2–3 minutes, until golden brown and cooked through. Remove the pancakes from the pan as soon as they are ready and keep them warm while you cook the remaining batter in the same way.

To serve, place a stack of pancakes on each plate and top with spoonfuls of the warm pears and the syrup.

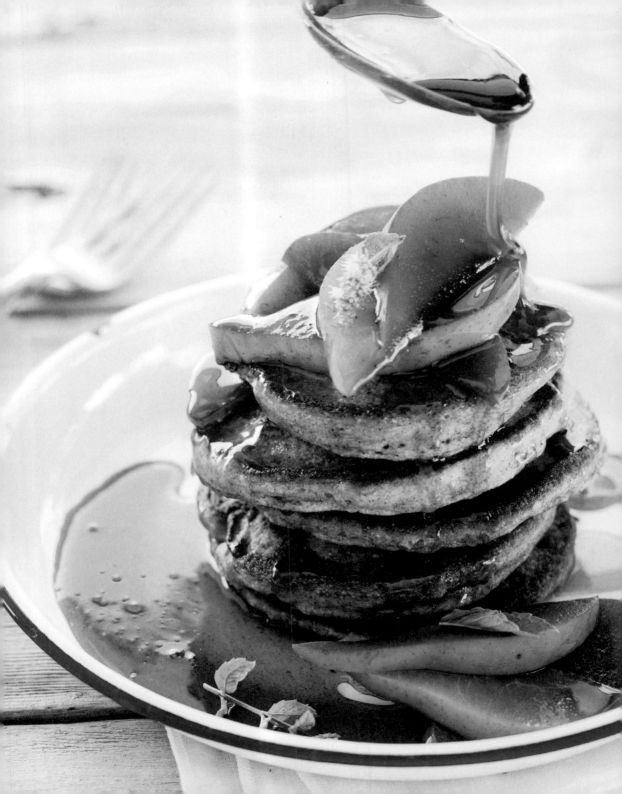

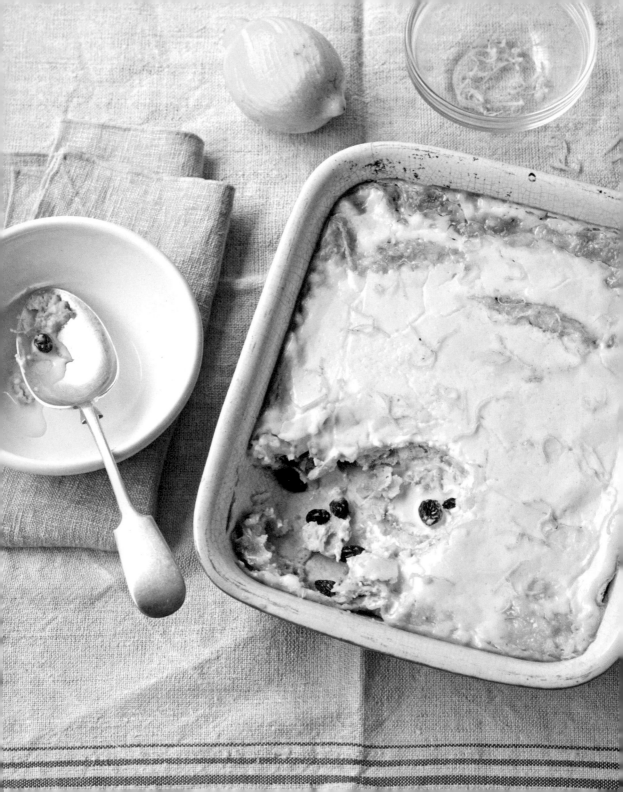

VEGAN BAKED LEMON PANCAKES

These pancakes are stuffed with a fragrant lemony filling made with blended non-dairy cream and tofu. These are then baked to create a light, creamy dessert that adults and kids alike will love.

PANCAKE BATTER

340 ml/1½ cups plain soy milk

¼ teaspoon salt

¼ teaspoon baking powder

grated zest of 1 lemon

215 g/1²/₃ cups unbleached plain/all-purpose flour

coconut or sunflower oil, for frying

LEMON FILLING

340 g/2 cups plain, firm tofu

685 ml/scant 3 cups thick soy or oat cream

pinch of salt

freshly squeezed juice of 2 lemons

grated zest of 3 lemons, plus extra to decorate

brown rice or agave syrup, to taste

30–60 g/¼–½ cup raisins (optional)

23 x 30 cm/9 x 12-inch baking pan or ovenproof dish, oiled

SERVES 4–6

For the pancakes, mix the milk and 225 ml/scant 1 cup water in a bowl. Stir in the salt, baking powder and lemon zest. Gradually add the flour, whisking vigorously until smooth. The batter should be thicker than conventional, egg-based pancake batter. Allow to rest for at least 15 minutes.

Heat a heavy-based frying pan/skillet and brush a little oil over it. When hot, pour a small ladleful of batter into the pan and tilt the pan to spread the batter evenly over the surface. Once the edges start turning golden brown, flip the pancake over and cook until golden on the reverse. Transfer to a plate, re-oil the pan and keep making pancakes in this way until all the batter is used up. Try to make the pancakes quite thin and that should give you 10 pancakes in total.

Preheat the oven to 130°C (350°F) Gas 4.

For the filling, put the tofu, 225 ml/scant 1 cup of the cream, the salt, lemon juice and zest and syrup, to taste, in a food processor and blend until smooth. Mix in the raisins: they give a lovely flavour to this dish, but you can omit them and add a little more syrup, if you wish.

Divide the filling between the pancakes, spreading it over each one. Roll the pancakes up tightly and arrange in the prepared baking pan or ovenproof dish. Pour the remaining cream evenly over the pancakes and decorate with some lemon zest.

Bake in the preheated oven for 15–20 minutes, until golden. Serve warm or cold.

VEGAN CRÊPES SUZETTE

This is a healthier version of the famous French dessert, Crêpes Suzette, made with agave syrup and coconut oil. These pancakes are egg-, sugar- and butter-free so the result is an irresistible vegan treat!

PANCAKE BATTER

165 ml/¾ cup soy milk

110 ml/⅓ cup plus 2 tablespoons water

¼ teaspoon bicarbonate of soda/baking soda

¼ teaspoon sea salt

130 g/1 cup unbleached plain/ all-purpose flour or millet flour

coconut oil, for frying

ORANGE GLAZE

8 tablespoons agave syrup

grated zest and freshly squeezed juice of 4 organic blood oranges or regular oranges

4 tablespoons extra virgin coconut oil, plus extra to finish

2–4 tablespoons rum (optional)

80 g/2¾ oz. dark/bittersweet vegan chocolate, to serve

SERVES 4

For the pancake batter, in a mixing bowl, combine the soy milk and water. Add the bicarbonate of soda/baking soda and salt. Slowly add the flour, whisking vigorously with a balloon whisk. The batter should be thicker than pancake batter made with eggs. Let it stand for at least 15 minutes.

Heat a frying pan/skillet and add a little coconut oil before pouring in the batter for each pancake. Pour a small ladleful of the batter into the pan and tilt the pan to spread the batter evenly over the surface. Once the edges start turning golden brown, flip the pancake over. Once golden on both sides, keep the pancake warm and cook the rest of the batter in the same way. The batter should make about eight medium pancakes.

For the orange glaze, heat half the agave syrup in a separate frying pan/ skillet over a medium heat until slightly caramelized. Add the remaining agave syrup and the orange zest and juice and bring to a slow boil. Add the coconut oil. The glaze shouldn't be too thick. At the end, add a little rum if you wish, for a richer aroma.

Pour most of the glaze from the pan into a bowl. Place a pancake in the pan and fold over twice to coat it well in the remaining glaze. Add more glaze for the second pancake and repeat until you use up all the pancakes. Serve the pancakes on a platter with any leftover glaze.

Melt the chocolate in a bowl set over a pan of barely simmering water, taking care that the base of the bowl does not touch the water. Stir in a few drops of coconut oil to make it glossy. Drizzle the chocolate over the pancakes just before serving.

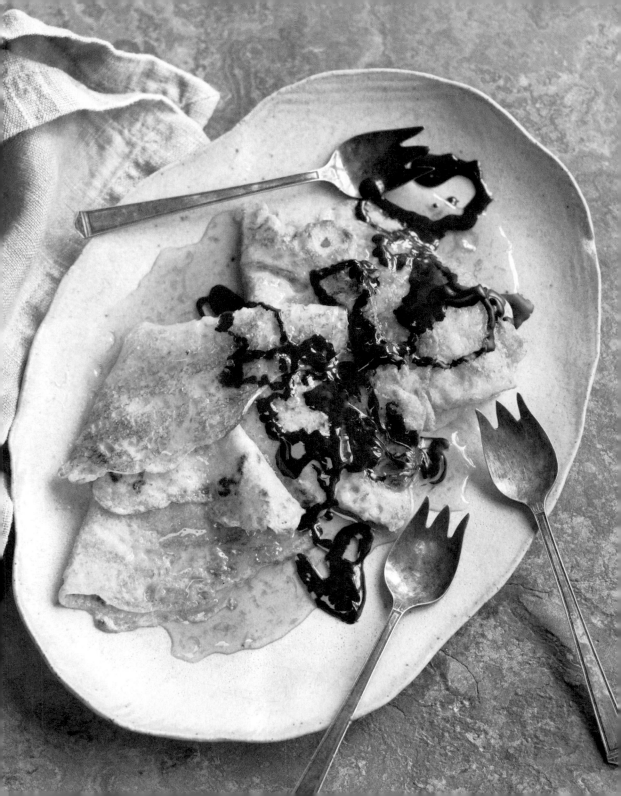

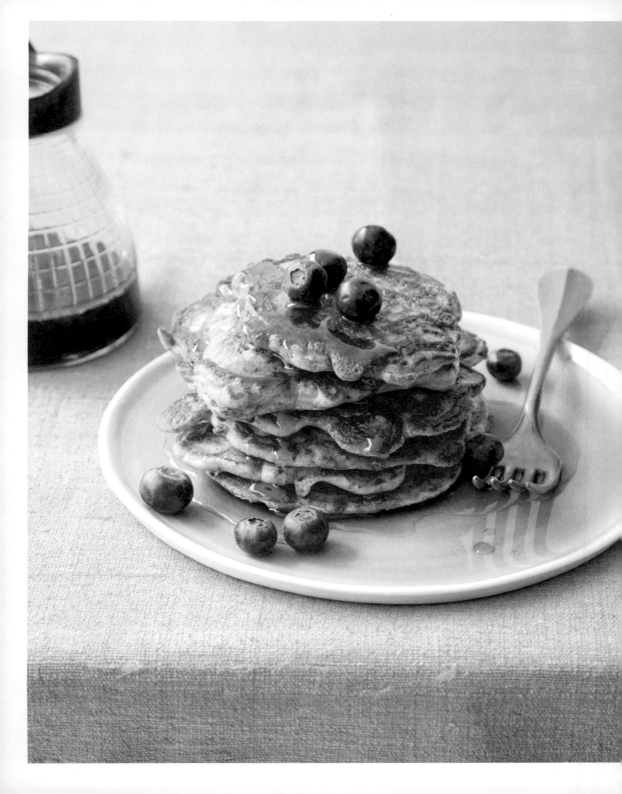

BUCKWHEAT & FLAXSEED PANCAKES

The nutrition factor is upped in these delicious American-style pancakes with the use of wholegrain flours and flaxseeds (linseeds), which are full of healthy fats, antioxidants and fibre. But don't skimp on the maple syrup – that's the best bit!

50 g/generous ⅓ cup potato starch

½ teaspoon bicarbonate of soda/baking soda

1½ teaspoons baking powder

70 g/½ cup buckwheat flour

60 g/scant ½ cup brown rice flour

3 tablespoons milled flaxseeds/ linseeds

½ teaspoon sea salt

1 teaspoon ground cinnamon

480 ml/2 cups almond milk

2 eggs (see Note)

1 teaspoon vanilla extract

vegetable oil, for frying

maple syrup, to taste

handful of blueberries, to serve (optional)

SERVES 2–4

Sift the potato starch, bicarbonate of soda/baking soda and baking powder into a mixing bowl. Add the remaining dry ingredients and set aside. In another bowl, combine the almond milk, eggs and vanilla extract. Add the wet into the dry ingredients gradually and whisk to make a thick batter.

Heat a little oil in a large frying pan/skillet over a medium-high heat. Drop the batter from a spoon into the pan to form six round circles. Cook until small bubbles form on the top of each pancake. Flip and cook for a further 3 minutes or until golden brown in colour.

Serve immediately, stacked on a plate and drizzled with maple syrup. Blueberries make a tasty addition, if desired, and are a powerful antioxidant.

Note: If you prefer not to use eggs, you could use egg replacer or make a flax-egg mix by combining 2 tablespoons of ground flaxseeds/linseeds with 6 tablespoons of water.

SPELT PANCAKES WITH FRIED BANANAS

These French-style thin pancakes are made with spelt flour, which is better for you than ordinary white flour with its high mineral and vitamin content. People with mild wheat intolerances also generally find they can tolerate spelt flour with no side effects.

sunflower oil, for frying

PANCAKE BATTER

100 g/¾ cup fine-grind spelt
   flour

½ teaspoon baking powder

pinch of sea salt

2 eggs

200 ml/generous ¾ cup
   rice milk

FRIED BANANAS

2 bananas, peeled

freshly squeezed juice
   of 1 orange

2 teaspoons agave syrup

1 teaspoon ground cinnamon

1 teaspoon desiccated/dried
   shredded coconut, plus extra
   to serve

MAKES ABOUT 5

To make the spelt pancakes, sift the flour, baking powder and salt into a large mixing bowl and make a well in the centre.

In a separate bowl, whisk together the eggs and milk. Gradually pour into the well in the flour mixture, mixing all the time until you get a smooth batter. Allow the batter to rest for at least 30 minutes. You can also make it the night before and keep it refrigerated if you are very organized.

When ready, heat a little oil in a non-stick frying pan/skillet until hot. Stir the batter and pour a small ladleful into the pan, swirling so that the mixture spreads to the edges. Cook until the top of the pancake starts to bubble – less than 1 minute – then flip it over and cook until golden. Remove the pancake from the pan as it's ready and keep warm while you cook the remaining batter in the same way.

To make the fried bananas, heat a little oil in a frying pan/skillet over a high heat. Slice the bananas and add to the hot pan. Fry until golden, then flip over and fry for another minute or so. Add the orange juice and agave syrup and dust the cinnamon and desiccated/dried shredded coconut over the top. Let the liquid bubble away for 30 seconds, then remove from the heat and transfer to a bowl.

Add some of the fried bananas to each pancake and fold it over into a parcel. Sprinkle over a little more coconut and enjoy immediately.

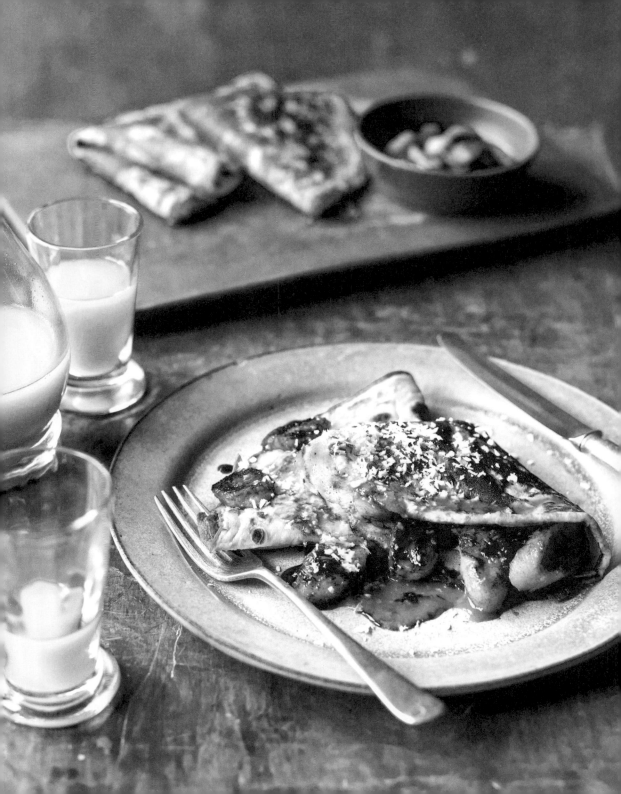

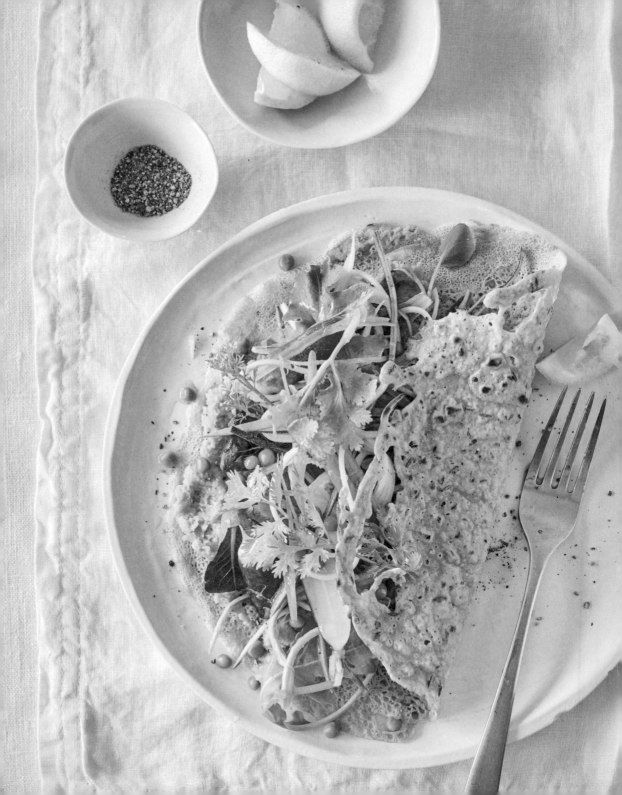

TURMERIC PANCAKES
WITH CARROT HUMMUS & VEGETABLES

Healthful turmeric, which contains antioxidant and anti-inflammatory properties, also adds savoury flavour and vivid colour to the batter for these pancakes. You can vary the filling by using whatever veggies are in season.

PANCAKE BATTER

2 teaspoons cumin seeds

150 g/1¼ cups chickpea (gram) flour

2 teaspoons ground turmeric

½ teaspoon salt

350 ml/1½ cups cold water

1 tablespoon olive oil, plus extra for frying

FILLING

500 g/18 oz. carrots, peeled and roughly chopped

1 tablespoon olive oil

200 g/7 oz. can chickpeas

1 small garlic clove, crushed

squeezed juice of 1 lemon

4 tablespoons extra virgin olive oil

¼ teaspoon ground cumin

1 cucumber, deseeded

1 large courgette/zucchini

1 bunch radishes

150 g/5½ oz. podded peas

100 g/3½ oz. salad leaves

handful of coriander/cilantro

extra oil, lemon juice and salt and pepper, to serve

MAKES 8 PANCAKES

Preheat the oven to 180°C (350°F) Gas 4 and line a roasting pan with baking parchment.

To make the carrot hummus place the carrots, olive oil, salt, pepper and 1 tablespoon of water into the prepared pan and roast in the preheated oven, covered with foil, for 40 minutes until tender. Set aside to cool. Reduce the oven to its lowest setting. Drain the chickpeas, reserving 3 tablespoons of their liquid. Purée the carrots, chickpeas and reserved liquid, garlic, half the lemon juice (reserving the rest for later), 3 tablespoons of the extra virgin olive oil, the cumin and some salt and pepper in a food processor until smooth. Set the hummus aside.

To make the pancakes, toast the cumin seeds in a dry frying pan/skillet until golden; let cool. Sift the chickpea (gram) flour, turmeric and salt into a bowl and stir in the cumin seeds. Make a well in the centre and beat in the water and oil to make a thin pouring batter. Rest for 15 minutes.

Meanwhile, thinly shred or slice the cucumber and courgette/zucchini. Halve or quarter the radishes. Blanch the peas in lightly salted boiling water for 2 minutes, drain, then refresh under cold water and pat dry. Combine the vegetables in a bowl and toss with the remaining lemon juice, remaining olive oil and some salt and pepper. Set aside.

Heat a frying pan/skillet over a medium heat. Drizzle with a little oil and then mop up with a paper towel. Pour in about 60 ml/¼ cup of the pancake mixture, swirling the pan to lightly coat the base. Cook over a medium-low heat for about 1½ minutes until the bottom is golden. Flip the pancake over and cook for a further 30–60 seconds until dotted with brown. Transfer to a low oven to keep warm. Repeat to make 8 pancakes.

To serve, spread a little carrot hummus onto each pancake, scatter over the shredded vegetables, the salad leaves and herbs. Wrap, roll, flip and serve drizzled with a little extra oil, lemon juice and black pepper.

GLUTEN-FREE SPINACH & RICOTTA CRÊPES

These delicate spinach crêpes are some of the best gluten-free pancakes you will ever try – the batter is much thinner than traditional crêpe batter and the overall effect is very light. Stuffed with ricotta, lemon and Parmesan, the flavours perfectly complement each other.

PANCAKE BATTER
80 g/²⁄₃ cup minus 1 tablespoon buckwheat flour, sifted

200 ml/generous ¾ cup water

2 eggs

1–2 tablespoons butter, for frying

SPINACH & RICOTTA FILLING
400 g/8 cups spinach, washed and drained

250 g/1 cup ricotta

pinch of freshly grated nutmeg

freshly squeezed juice of 1 lemon plus 1 teaspoon of the grated zest

sea salt and freshly ground black pepper

60 g/scant 1 cup grated Parmesan cheese, plus extra to serve

crêpe swizzle stick (optional)

SERVES 6

Begin by preparing the filling. Bring a saucepan of water to the boil over a high heat and season with salt. Add the spinach to the pan and cook in the water for a few minutes until it is just wilted but still vibrant green. Drain and immediately plunge the spinach into cold water. Once cool, put the spinach in a clean kitchen cloth, fold up tightly and squeeze out as much water as possible. Remove a third of the spinach and purée in a food processor with 1 tablespoon of water. Set the purée aside until you are ready to cook the crêpes.

Finely chop the remaining spinach and mix together with the ricotta. Season with salt and pepper, the nutmeg and the lemon juice and zest. Fold in the Parmesan, then store in the refrigerator.

To make the crêpe batter, put the flour, water, eggs and reserved spinach purée into a large mixing bowl. Season with salt and pepper and whisk until you have a smooth and runny batter. Cover and put the batter in the refrigerator to rest for 30 minutes.

When you are ready to serve, remove the batter from the refrigerator and stir gently. Put a little butter in a large frying pan/skillet set over a medium heat. Allow the butter to melt and coat the base of the pan, then ladle a spoonful of the rested batter into the pan and quickly spread the batter out very thinly. You can do this either by tilting the pan, or, for best results, use a crêpe swizzle stick. Cook until the top of the pancake is set, then turn over carefully with a spatula and cook on the other side for a further 1–2 minutes until the crêpe is crispy. Keep the crêpe warm while you cook the remaining batter in the same way.

Put some of the chilled ricotta filling in the centre of each crêpe and roll up to serve. Top with a little extra grated Parmesan, if desired. Serve.

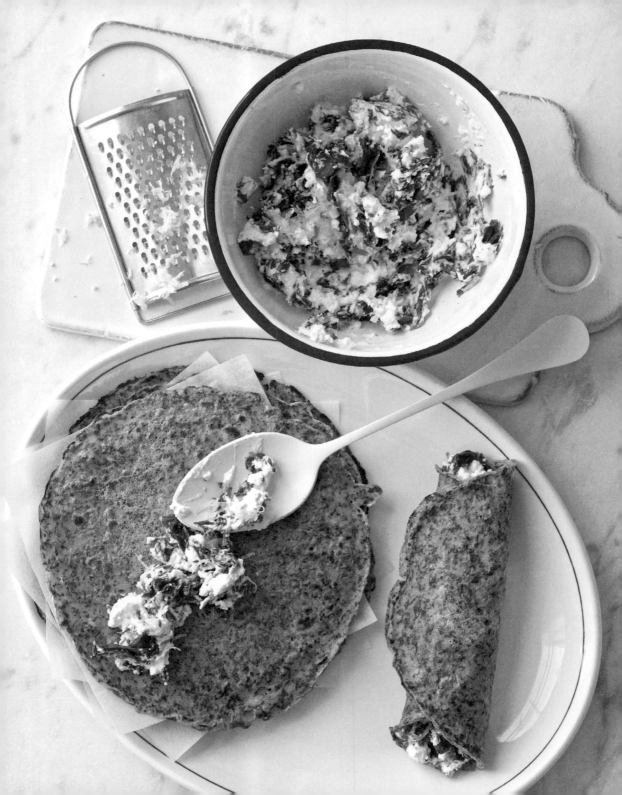

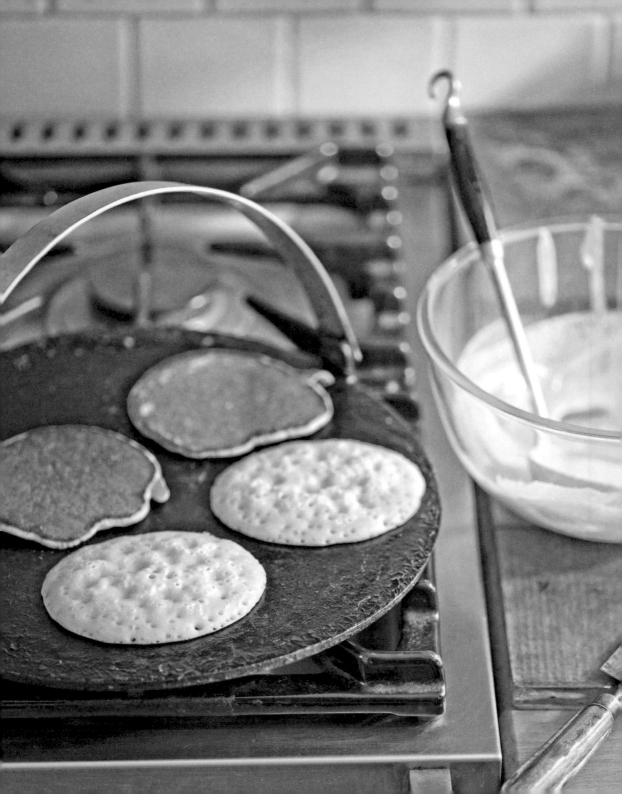

POSH PANCAKES

BEETROOT PANCAKES WITH GOAT'S CHEESE, ONION RELISH & WALNUTS

PANCAKE BATTER

2 eggs

220 ml/scant 1 cup whole milk

75 g/½ cup plus 1 tablespoon plain/all-purpose flour

25 g/3 tablespoons rye flour

pinch of salt

55 g/2 oz. cooked beetroot/beet, finely chopped

1 tablespoons olive oil, plus extra for frying

FILLING

300 g/10½ oz. frozen spinach, thawed

300 g/10½ oz. soft goat's cheese

2 tablespoons freshly chopped basil

50 g/⅓ cup chopped walnuts

6 tablespoons grated Parmesan cheese

ONION RELISH

2 tablespoons olive oil

3 onions, thinly sliced

2 tablespoons balsamic vinegar

2 tablespoons soft brown sugar

sea salt and freshly ground black pepper

rocket/arugula, fresh basil leaves and Parmesan shavings, to serve

MAKES 16 PANCAKES

The beetroot/beet adds attractive colour to these savoury pancakes, as well as a hint of earthy flavour. A little rye flour is used in the batter here too for its deep, strong taste, but it can be easily replaced with plain/all-purpose flour.

Start by making the onion relish. Heat the olive oil in a saucepan over a low-medium heat. Add the onions and a little salt and pepper and cook for 20 minutes, stirring occasionally, until they are really soft and golden. Add the vinegar and sugar and cook for a further 5–10 minutes until jammy in consistency. Leave to cool.

To make the pancakes, place the eggs, half the milk, the flours, salt and chopped beetroot/beet in a food processor and blend until the beetroot/beet is puréed and the mixture is smooth. Add the remaining milk and the oil and blend again. Transfer to a jug/pitcher and leave to rest for 20 minutes.

Meanwhile, make the filling. Squeeze out all the excess water from the thawed spinach and chop finely. Place in a bowl and beat in the goat's cheese, basil, walnuts and grated Parmesan. Season to taste with salt and pepper.

Lightly stir the pancake mixture once. Heat a frying pan/skillet over a medium heat, brush with oil and swirl in about 60 ml/¼ cup of the pancake mixture, making sure it covers the base. Cook over a medium-low heat for about 1½ minutes until the base is golden. Flip the pancake over and cook for a further 1 minute until dotted brown. Remove the pancake from the pan as soon as it is ready and keep warm while you cook the remaining batter in the same way.

When you are ready to serve, spoon the goat's cheese mixture down the centre of each pancake. Top with a few rocket/arugula leaves, fresh basil leaves and a spoonful of the onion relish. Roll up and enjoy. Serve the pancakes with extra relish and shavings of Parmesan cheese.

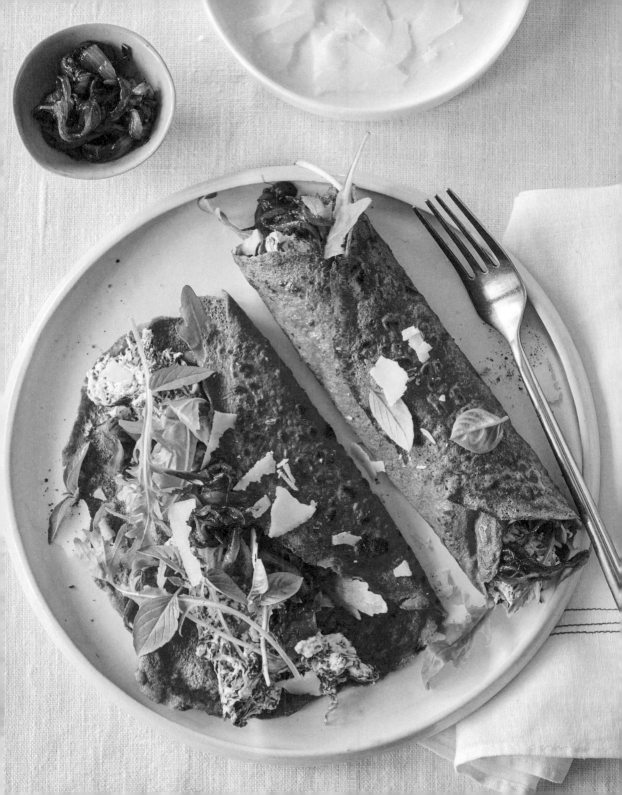

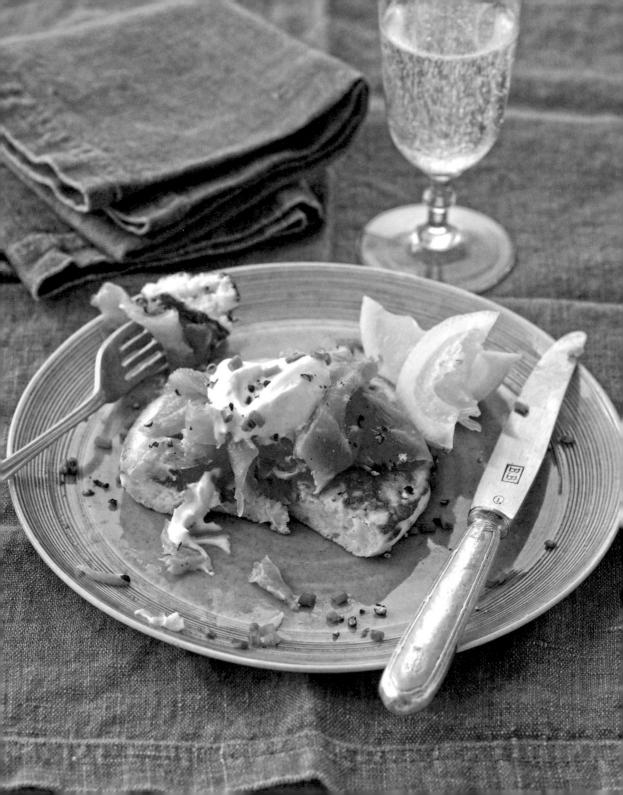

BUTTERMILK PANCAKES
WITH SALMON & HORSERADISH CREAM

Bellini pancakes topped with smoked salmon make fantastic canapés. For a more indulgent version, why not serve large, fluffy buttermilk pancakes seasoned with chives and topped with thick slices of smoked salmon and horseradish cream? This is great as a brunch dish or a light lunch.

170 g/1¼ cups self-raising/ rising flour, sifted

1 teaspoon baking powder

2 eggs, separated

200 ml/generous ¾ cup buttermilk

2 teaspoons caster/ granulated sugar

1 tablespoon freshly chopped chives, plus extra for sprinkling

100 ml/⅓ cup plus 1 tablespoon whole milk

250 ml/1 cup plus 1 tablespoon crème fraîche

1 heaped tablespoon creamed horseradish

1–2 tablespoons butter, for frying

sea salt and freshly ground black pepper

400 g/2½ cups smoked salmon slices, to serve

1 lemon, sliced into wedges, to serve

SERVES 4

To make the pancake batter, put the flour, baking powder, egg yolks, buttermilk, caster/granulated sugar and chives in a large mixing bowl and whisk together. Season well with salt and pepper, then gradually add the milk until the batter is smooth and pourable.

In a separate bowl, whisk the egg whites to stiff peaks. Gently fold the whisked egg whites into the batter mixture using a spatula. Cover and put in the refrigerator to rest for 30 minutes.

For the horseradish cream, whisk together the crème fraîche and horseradish in a small bowl and season with salt and pepper.

When you are ready to serve, remove the batter mixture from the refrigerator and stir once. Put a little butter in a large frying pan/skillet set over a medium heat. Allow the butter to melt and coat the base of the pan, then ladle small amounts of the batter into the pan, leaving a little space between each. Cook until the underside of each pancake is golden brown and a few bubbles start to appear on the top – this will take about 2–3 minutes. Turn the pancakes over using a spatula and cook on the other side until golden brown. Remove the pancakes from the pan as they are ready and keep them warm while you cook the remaining batter in the same way, adding more butter as needed.

Serve the pancakes warm, topped with a generous spoonful of the horseradish cream, slices of smoked salmon and wedges of lemon to squeeze over the top. Sprinkle with extra chopped chives and enjoy.

SQUASH & GOAT'S CHEESE PANCAKES

Perfect for a sophisticated lunch, these pancakes are topped with sour/
soured cream or crème fraîche and drizzled with delicious pumpkin seed oil.
Use a mild, creamy goat's cheese so that the flavour is not overpowering
when combined with the delicately spiced butternut squash.

1 butternut squash, peeled and
seeds removed (670 g/1½ lb),
diced

2 tablespoons olive oil

1 teaspoon black onion seeds

pinch of spiced sea salt or
regular sea salt

4–5 curry leaves, crushed

1–2 garlic cloves, skins on

200 g/1½ cups self-raising/
rising flour, sifted

2 teaspoons baking powder

1 egg

300 ml/1¼ cups whole milk

3 tablespoons melted butter,
plus extra for greasing

125 g/1 cup soft goat's cheese

sour/soured cream or crème
fraîche, to serve

bunch of fresh Greek basil
leaves, to garnish

pumpkin seed oil, to drizzle

sea salt and freshly ground
black pepper

ovenproof roasting pan, greased

SERVES 4

Preheat the oven to 180°C (350°F) Gas 4.

Put the diced butternut squash in the prepared roasting pan. Drizzle with
the oil and sprinkle over the onion seeds, salt and curry leaves. Stir to coat
the squash in the oil and spices, then add the garlic cloves to the pan.
Roast in the preheated oven for 35–45 minutes until the squash is soft
and starts to caramelize at the edges. Leave to cool completely.

To make the pancake batter, put the flour, baking powder, egg and milk in
a large mixing bowl and whisk together. Season with salt and pepper.
Add the melted butter and whisk again. The batter should have a smooth,
dropping consistency. Add about two-thirds of the butternut squash to
the batter and set aside.

Remove the skins from the garlic cloves and mash to a paste using a fork.
Whisk into the batter, then crumble in the goat's cheese. Mix together
gently. Cover and put in the refrigerator to rest for 30 minutes.

Put a little butter in a large frying pan/skillet set over a medium heat.
Allow the butter to melt and coat the base of the pan, then ladle spoonfuls
of the rested batter into the pan, leaving a little space between each.

Cook until the underside of each pancake is golden brown and a few
bubbles start to appear on the top – this will take about 2–3 minutes.
Turn the pancakes over using a spatula and cook on the other side until
golden brown. Remove the pancakes from the pan as they are ready and
keep them warm while you cook the remaining batter in the same way.

Serve the pancakes, topped with a spoonful of sour/soured cream or
crème fraîche, a few sprigs of basil and the reserved butternut squash.
Drizzle with pumpkin seed oil and sprinkle with ground black pepper.

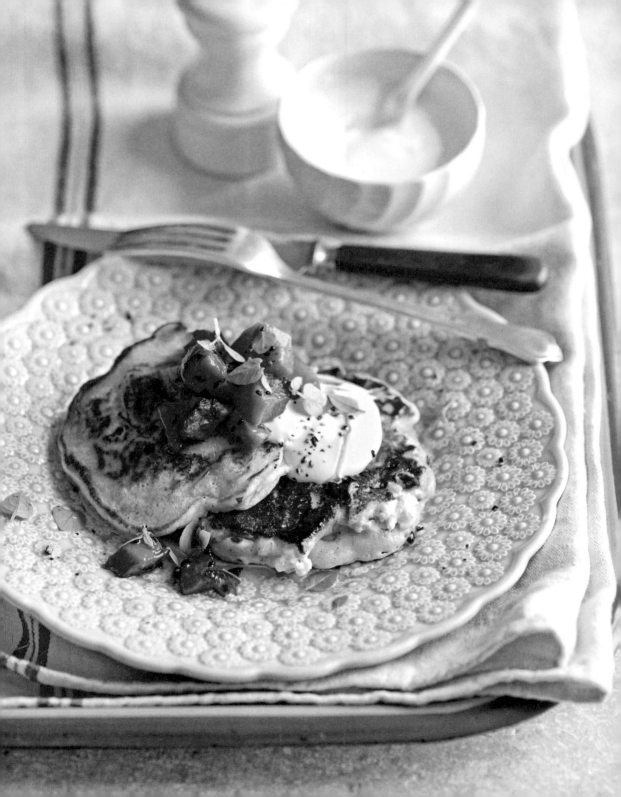

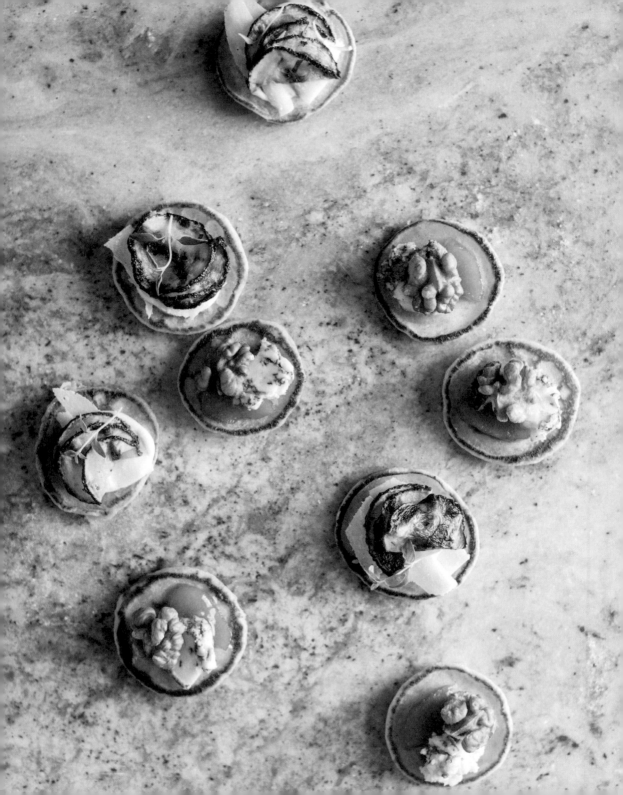

BLINIS WITH COURGETTE & PARMESAN & PEAR PURÉE, BLUE CHEESE & WALNUTS

This blini recipe makes about 70 mini pancakes. You can use a squeezy bottle if you want neat circles or use two teaspoons for a more rustic look.

PANCAKE BATTER

40 g/generous ¼ cup spelt flour

130 g/1 cup minus 1 tablespoon white/strong bread flour

1 teaspoon salt

1 x 7 g/¼ oz. sachet easy blend/ rapid-rise dried yeast

150 ml/⅔ cup crème fraîche or sour/soured cream

175 ml/¾ cup whole milk

2 eggs, separated

30 g/2 tablespoons butter

COURGETTE TOPPING

2 courgettes/zucchini

100 g/3½ oz. Parmesan

grated zest of ½ lemon

1 garlic clove, crushed

1 tablespoon fresh thyme leaves

4 tablespoons olive oil

sea salt and black pepper

MAKES 40 TOPPINGS

PEAR & BLUE CHEESE TOPPING

3 ripe Williams/Comice pears

squeezed juice of 1 lemon

100 g/3½ oz. blue cheese

30 walnut halves

MAKES 30 TOPPINGS

For the pancake batter, sift together the flours and salt and sprinkle over the yeast. In a small saucepan, warm the crème fraîche or sour cream and milk. When just warm (not hot) to the touch, whisk in the egg yolks. Pour the mixture over the flour and yeast. Mix well, cover with a kitchen cloth and leave in a warm place for 1 hour.

In a separate clean bowl, whisk the egg whites until they form stiff peaks, then gently fold into the batter.

Heat a non-stick frying pan/skillet and rub the base with butter using a paper towel. In batches, spoon teaspoons of batter into the pan or use a squeezy bottle to make 4-cm/1½-inch blinis. When tiny bubbles appear on top, use a palette knife to flip each pancake and cook briefly on the other side. Leave to cool on a wire rack while you use up the rest of the batter, then serve with your desired toppings.

For the courgette/zucchini topping. Slice the courgettes/zucchini into 2-mm/¹⁄₁₆-inch slices. Using a vegetable peeler, peel 40 strips of Parmesan and place one each on top of 40 blinis. Set aside.

Mix the lemon zest, garlic and thyme into the oil, season with salt and pepper, and toss through the courgettes/zucchini.

Heat a large ridged griddle pan/grill pan over a medium heat. Place the courgette/zucchini slices onto the hot grill and cook for 1 minute, then flip over with tongs. When the edges start to crisp, transfer two slices of courgette/zucchini onto each of the 40 blinis, then serve.

For the pear purée and blue cheese topping, peel, core and dice the pears and put them in a non-stick pan with the lemon juice. Cook over a medium heat, stirring constantly for around 20 minutes, until you have a thick but loose paste. Let the pear purée cool.

Top each of the 30 blinis with a little pear purée, blue cheese and a walnut half, then serve. The pear purée will keep for up to 1 week stored in an airtight container in the refrigerator.

KIMCHI PANCAKE
WITH BLACK GARLIC CRÈME FRAÎCHE

This take on this popular Korean dish contrasts the chewy-textured, chilli/chile-hot pancake with the subtle coolness of crème fraîche, enriched with the mellow sweetness of black garlic. Kimchi is a traditional Korean fermented relish, usually made with cabbage.

100 g/³⁄₄ cup plain/
  all-purpose flour

½ teaspoon salt

3 tablespoons kimchi liquid
  (reserved from kimchi)

130 g/1 cup kimchi, finely
  chopped

1 spring onion/scallion, finely
  chopped

150 ml/²⁄₃ cup crème fraîche or
  sour/soured cream

3 black garlic cloves, finely
  chopped

1 tablespoon sunflower
  or vegetable oil

thinly sliced spring onion/
  scallion, to garnish

SERVES 2

Make the batter by whisking together the flour and salt with 100 ml/ ¹⁄₃ cup plus 1 tablespoon water into a thick paste. Stir in the kimchi liquid, then mix in the kimchi and spring onion/scallion.

Mix together the crème fraîche or sour/soured cream and black garlic and set aside.

Heat a large frying pan/skillet until hot. Add the oil and heat well. Pour in the batter, which should sizzle as it hits the pan, spreading it to form an even layer. Fry for 3–5 minutes until set, then turn over and fry the pancake for a further 3–4 minutes until it is well browned on both sides. Remove the pancake from the pan to a plate.

Cut the kimchi pancake into portions and serve topped with the black garlic crème fraîche or sour/soured cream. Sprinkle with extra spring onion/scallion to garnish.

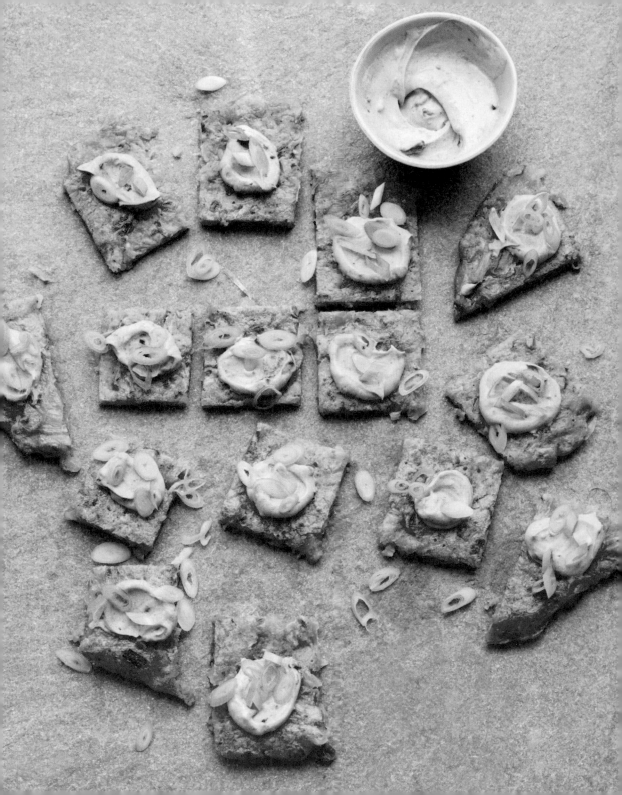

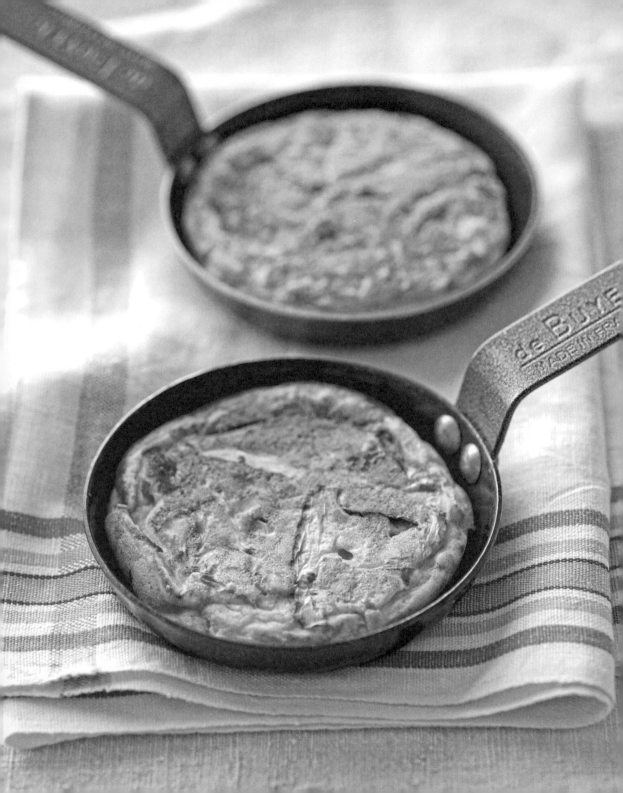

COURGETTE & FETA PANCAKES

These pancakes are quick and easy to prepare and make a great accompaniment to soups as an alternative to bread. The feta cheese melts when cooked, giving them a lovely soft texture. This recipe uses raw courgette/zucchini, but if you prefer, you can fry it until soft in a little olive oil before adding to the pancake batter. Just make sure that you drain the courgette/zucchini of its cooking juices and let it cool first.

150 g/1 cup plus 2 tablespoons self-raising/rising flour, sifted

2 eggs, separated

250 ml/1 cup plus 1 tablespoon whole milk

70 g/⅓ cup minus 1 teaspoon butter, melted and cooled, plus extra for frying

1 teaspoon baking powder

1 large grated courgette/ zucchini (approx. 200 g/ 2½ cups)

200 g/1½ cups feta cheese, crumbled

1 tablespoon freshly chopped mint

sea salt and freshly ground black pepper

MAKES 10

To make the pancake batter, put the flour, egg yolks, milk, melted butter and baking powder in a large mixing bowl and whisk together. Season well with salt and pepper and mix again until you have a smooth batter.

In a separate bowl, whisk the egg whites to stiff peaks. Gently fold the whisked egg whites into the batter mixture using a spatula. Cover and put in the refrigerator to rest for 30 minutes.

When you are ready to serve, remove the batter mixture from the refrigerator and stir gently. Add the grated courgette/zucchini to the batter with the feta cheese and mint.

Put a little butter in a large frying pan/skillet set over a medium heat (alternatively, you can use small individual frying pans/skillets if you have them). Allow the butter to melt and coat the base of the pan, then ladle small amounts of the rested batter into the pan, leaving a little space between each. Cook until the underside of each pancake is golden brown and a few bubbles start to appear on the top – this will take about 2–3 minutes. Turn the pancakes over using a spatula and cook on the other side until golden brown. It is important that they cook all the way through to ensure that the middle of your pancakes are not soggy.

Serve immediately.

SOCCA PANCAKES
WITH ROASTED PEARS & TAHINI DRIZZLE

Socca are gluten-free pancakes made with protein-rich chickpea (gram) flour which makes them extra satisfying. This pear and maple-tahini topping is also good served with yogurt, ice cream or waffles. Both the pears and the sauce can be made in advance and the pears can be warmed up before topping the socca.

PANCAKE BATTER
125 g/1 cup minus 1 tablespoon chickpea (gram) flour
½ teaspoon salt
olive oil or butter, for frying

ROASTED PEARS
melted coconut oil, for brushing
2 firm pears (such as Bosc) cored and sliced lengthways into 5 mm/¼-inch thick slices
¼ teaspoon ground cinnamon, plus more if needed

MAPLE-TAHINI DRIZZLE
60 g/¼ cup tahini
60 ml/¼ cup almond milk
1–2 tablespoons maple syrup
¼ teaspoon ground cinnamon
¼ teaspoon vanilla extract

baking sheet, lined with baking parchment

SERVES 2

For the pancake batter, put the chickpea (gram) flour, salt and 295 ml/ 1¼ cups water into a large bowl and mix together with a whisk or a fork until well combined into a smooth batter. Leave to stand at room temperature for at least 10 minutes.

Preheat the oven to 180°C (350°F) Gas 4.

For the roasted pears, brush the baking parchment on the baking sheet with melted coconut oil and arrange the pear slices on top in a single layer. Brush the pears with more melted coconut oil and then sprinkle with cinnamon. Bake in the preheated oven for 30–40 minutes, flipping them at the 20-minute mark, until the pears have softened and are beginning to turn golden.

Meanwhile, prepare the maple-tahini drizzle. In a small bowl or jar, combine the tahini, almond milk, maple syrup, cinnamon and vanilla. Whisk by hand or use a stick blender to blend together until smooth.

Heat a little olive oil or butter in another small frying pan/skillet over a medium heat. Add approximately 60–75 ml/¼ – scant ⅓ cup of the socca batter to the warm pan. Swirl it around so that it covers the base of the pan. Fry for about 2–3 minutes, until the batter begins to form bubbles. Flip the pancake with a spatula and cook for another 1–2 minutes on the other side. Remove the pancake from the pan as soon it is ready and keep warm while you cook the remaining batter in the same way. This should make you about four small socca pancakes in total.

Top the warm socca pancakes with the maple-tahini drizzle and pears and serve.

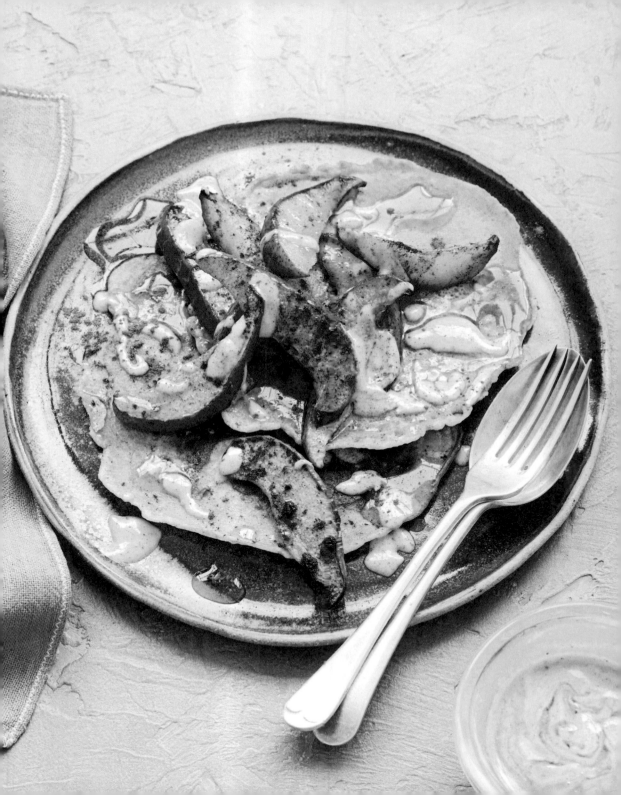

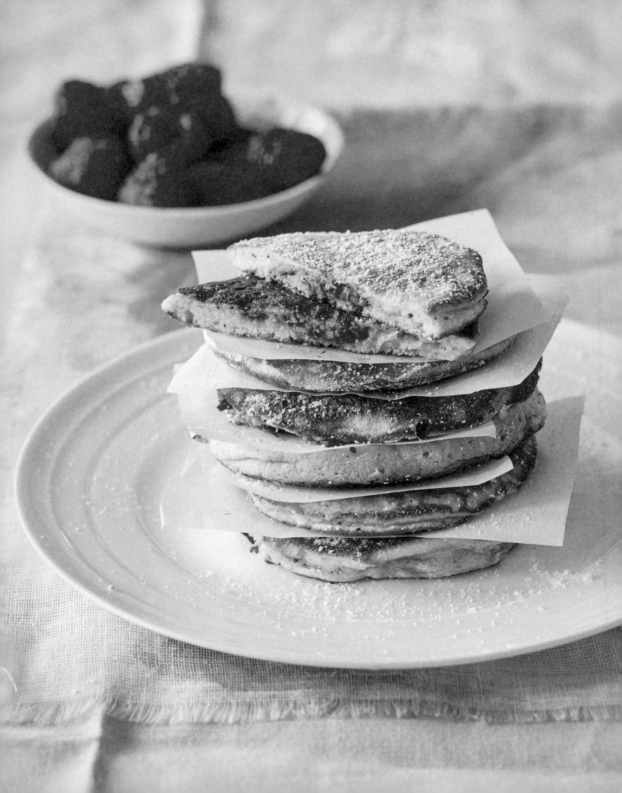

POPPY SEED PANCAKES STUFFED WITH CRUSHED CINNAMON RASPBERRIES

The best method with these fancy pancakes is to pour in the batter and once the top is almost set, add your raspberry mixture, then spoon over more batter and carefully spread this over the filling. Allow a few seconds before flipping over to cook the second side of each. They can be tricky to master at first but are worth a little effort.

RASPBERRY FILLING

100 g/scant 1 cup fresh raspberries, plus extra to serve

1 tablespoon caster/granulated sugar

¼ teaspoon ground cinnamon

PANCAKE BATTER

60 g/scant ½ cup self raising/ rising flour

1 teaspoon baking powder

2 eggs, separated

50 ml/3½ tablespoons buttermilk

1 tablespoon melted butter

¼ teaspoon vanilla extract

2 teaspoons poppy seeds

25 g/2 tablespoons caster/ granulated sugar

vegetable oil, for frying

icing/confectioners' sugar, to serve

MAKES 8

Begin by making the raspberry filling. Place the raspberries, sugar and cinnamon in a bowl and mash with a fork. Leave to marinate for 10 minutes, then strain and discard the juices. Set the crushed cinnamon raspberries aside.

Meanwhile, to make the pancakes, sift together the flour and baking powder. In a bowl beat the egg yolks, buttermilk, butter and vanilla and then whisk in the flour and baking powder. Fold in the poppy seeds.

In a separate bowl using a hand-held electric whisk, beat the egg whites and sugar together for 2–3 minutes until stiff peaks form. Stir a third of the mixture through the batter and then carefully fold in the rest until evenly combined.

Heat a frying pan/skillet over a low heat and brush with vegetable oil. Pour about 30 ml/2 tablespoons of the batter into the pan (two portions at a time) and cook over a medium-low heat for 1 minute. Carefully spread 2 teaspoons of the crushed raspberry mixture in the centre of each pancake and as soon as the edges of the pancakes are starting to set, spoon over enough of the batter to coat the filling.

Continue cooking the pancakes for a further 1 minute until almost set, then flip over and cook for a further 30 seconds or until golden underneath and set. Remove the pancakes from the pan and keep them warm while you cook the remaining batter in the same way.

Dust the pancakes with icing/confectioners' sugar and serve with a few fresh raspberries.

SOUFFLÉ PANCAKES
WITH COCONUT CREAM & PASSION FRUIT SYRUP

A different take on the usual French or American-style pancakes, these Japanese-style soufflé pancakes are super light and fluffy. The batter is cooked in crumpet rings or in cookie cutters, whichever you have to hand, but remember to oil them well each time between pancakes.

PANCAKE BATTER

60 g/scant ½ cup self-raising/ rising flour

1 teaspoon baking powder

2 eggs, separated

40 ml/2¾ tablespoons milk

1 tablespoon melted butter

¼ teaspoon vanilla extract

45 g/3½ tablespoons caster/ granulated sugar

vegetable oil, for greasing

PASSION FRUIT SYRUP

100 ml/⅓ cup plus 1 tablespoon passion fruit pulp

50 g/¼ cup caster/granulated sugar

COCONUT CREAM

50 ml/3½ tablespoons whipping cream

2 tablespoons coconut cream

1 tablespoon caster/granulated sugar

icing/confectioners' sugar and toasted coconut, to serve

2 x 10-cm/4-inch crumpet rings or cookie cutters

MAKES 6

Begin by making the passion fruit syrup. Place the passion fruit pulp, sugar and 50 ml/3½ tablespoons water in a small saucepan and heat gently, stirring, to dissolve the sugar. Simmer for 10 minutes or until it is syrup-like. Set aside to cool.

For the coconut cream, whip the cream until it's starting to hold its shape, then whisk in the coconut cream and sugar. Chill until required.

For the pancakes, sift together the flour and baking powder. In a separate bowl, beat the egg yolks, milk, melted butter and vanilla extract together and then whisk in the flour and baking powder. In a separate bowl using a hand-held electric whisk, beat the egg whites and sugar together for 2–3 minutes until stiff peaks form. Stir a third of the mixture through the batter and then carefully fold in the rest until evenly combined.

Oil the insides of the crumpet rings or cookie cutters and lightly oil a pancake pan. Place the pan over a medium heat and place the two oiled rings in the pan.

Spoon about 50 ml/3½ tablespoons of the pancake batter into each ring so that it comes about two-thirds of the way up the sides. Add 2 tablespoons of water to the pan around the edge and cover with a lid or upside-down pan. Cook over a medium heat for 2–3 minutes until the pancakes are almost set. Flip the rings over and cook the second side of the pancakes for a further 1 minute until lightly browned and the pancakes are set through. Remove from the pan and then carefully press the pancakes out of their rings. Keep them warm while you cook the remaining batter in the same way.

Dust the pancakes with icing/confectioners' sugar, top with toasted coconut and serve drizzled with passion fruit syrup and coconut cream.

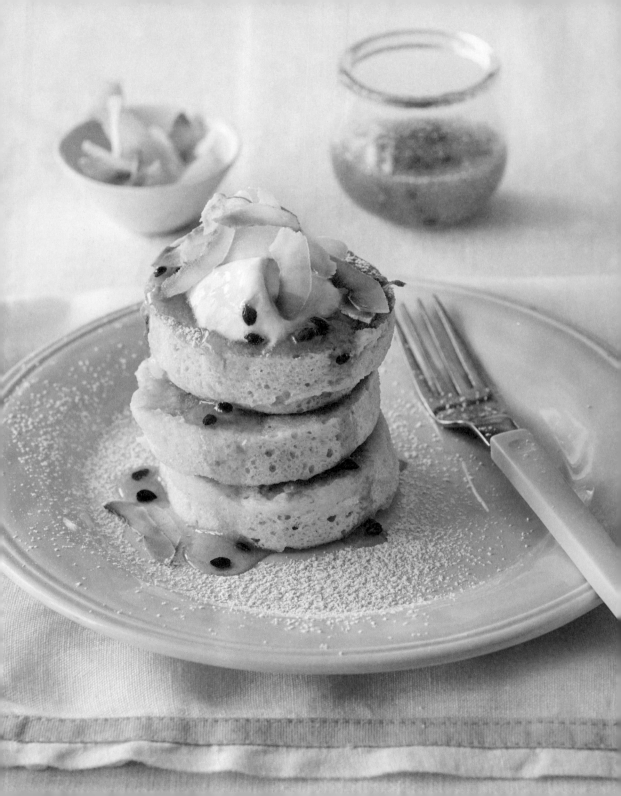

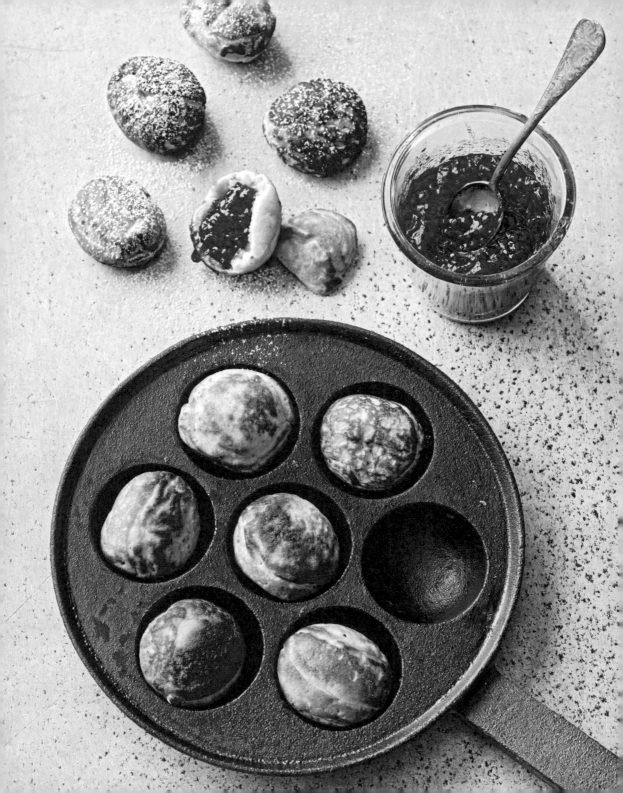

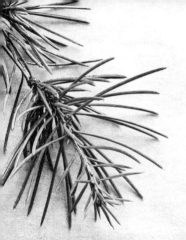

DANISH CHRISTMAS PANCAKES

Go to any Danish household in December, and you are likely to be served these festive little treats. They are traditionally sometimes baked with a little piece of apple inside each, which you can add, if you like.

3 eggs, separated

300 ml/1¼ cups buttermilk

100 ml/⅓ cup plus 1 tablespoon double/heavy cream

1 teaspoon vanilla extract

1 tablespoon caster/granulated sugar

½ teaspoon salt

1 teaspoon baking powder

½ teaspoon bicarbonate of soda/baking soda

250 g/1¾ cups plus 2 tablespoons plain/ all-purpose flour

1 teaspoon ground cardamom

grated zest of 1 medium lemon (or to taste)

50 g/3½ tablespoons butter, melted, for frying

icing/confectioners' sugar, to serve

raspberry jam/jelly, for dipping (optional)

an aebleskiver pan, Japanese takoyaki pan or frying pan/ skillet

MAKES 30

Mix together the egg yolks, buttermilk, double/heavy cream and vanilla extract in a large mixing bowl. In a separate bowl, sift together all the dry ingredients including the cardamom.

In another clean bowl, whisk the egg whites until stiff using a hand-held electric whisk.

Add the egg and cream mixture to the dry ingredients, then carefully fold in the beaten egg whites and lemon zest. Leave to rest for 30 minutes in the refrigerator before using.

Place the pan over a high heat to warm through and add a little melted butter to the pan to stop the pancakes from sticking. If you are using an aebleskiver pan, carefully add enough batter to each hole so that it reaches about 3 mm/⅛ inch from the top. If you are using a normal frying pan/skillet, add spoonfuls of batter as you would if making normal small pancakes. Leave to cook for a few minutes until the edges become firm then, using a fork or knitting needle (knitting needle is easier!), gently turn the pancakes over to cook on the other side.

Once browned on both sides (3–4 minutes per batch), keep the cooked pancakes warm until you have finished frying.

Serve the pancakes dusted with icing/confectioners' sugar and a little pot of raspberry jam/jelly for dipping.

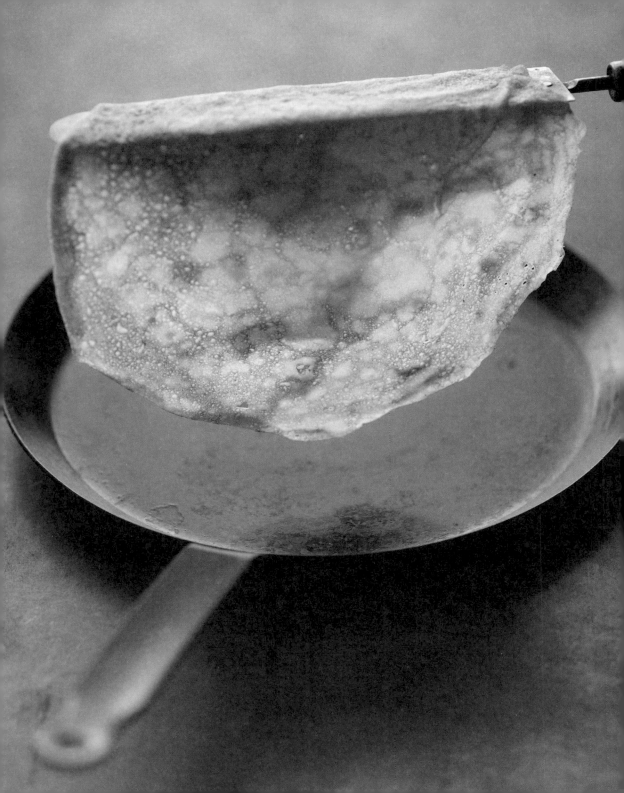

SWEET &
STICKY

OREO PANCAKES
WITH CHOCOLATE FUDGE SAUCE

PANCAKE BATTER

160 g/scant 1¼ cups self-raising/rising flour, sifted

1 teaspoon baking powder

1 egg, separated

1 teaspoon vanilla extract

2 tablespoons caster/granulated sugar

pinch of salt

250 ml/1 cup plus 1 tablespoon whole milk

2 tablespoons melted butter, plus extra for frying

9 Oreo cookies or similar, broken into pieces

CHOCOLATE FUDGE SAUCE

30 g/⅓ cup cocoa powder, sifted

1 teaspoon cold water

150 ml/⅔ cup double/heavy cream

100 g/⅓ cup milk/semi-sweet chocolate, chopped

1 tablespoon golden/light corn syrup

1 tablespoon butter

pinch of salt

1 teaspoon vanilla extract

MAKES 12

The Oreo pieces in these pancakes soften when cooked, creating delicious chocolate bursts. Served with a wickedly sweet chocolate sauce, these are definitely pancakes for a special treat rather than every day.

To make the pancake batter, put the flour, baking powder, egg yolk, vanilla, sugar, salt and milk into a large mixing bowl and whisk together. Add the melted butter and whisk again. The batter should have a smooth, dropping consistency.

In a separate bowl, whisk the egg white to stiff peaks. Gently fold the whisked egg white into the batter mixture using a spatula. Cover and put in the refrigerator to rest for 30 minutes.

For the chocolate fudge sauce, mix the cocoa powder with the cold water until you have a smooth paste. Put the cream, chocolate, cocoa paste, golden/light corn syrup, butter, salt and vanilla extract in a saucepan set over a medium heat and simmer until the chocolate has melted and you have a smooth, glossy sauce. Keep the pan over a low heat to keep the sauce warm until you are ready to serve.

When you are ready to serve, remove your batter mixture from the refrigerator and stir once. Put a little butter in a large frying pan/skillet set over a medium heat. Allow the butter to melt and coat the base of the pan, then ladle small amounts of the batter into the pan. Sprinkle some of the Oreo cookies into the batter and cook until the batter is just set, then turn over and cook for a further 2–3 minutes. Once cooked, keep the pancakes warm while you cook the remaining batter in the same way, adding a little butter to the pan each time, if required.

Serve the pancakes in stacks with the hot chocolate fudge sauce poured over the top.

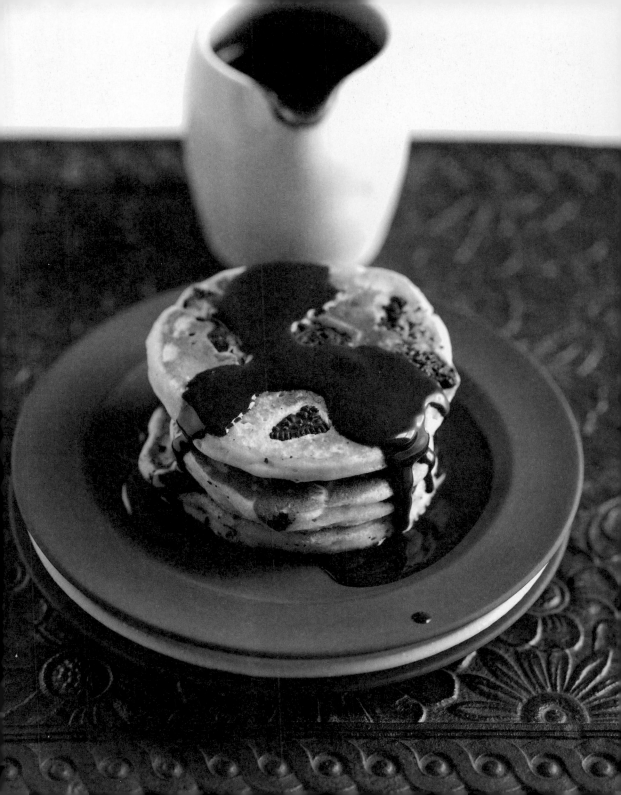

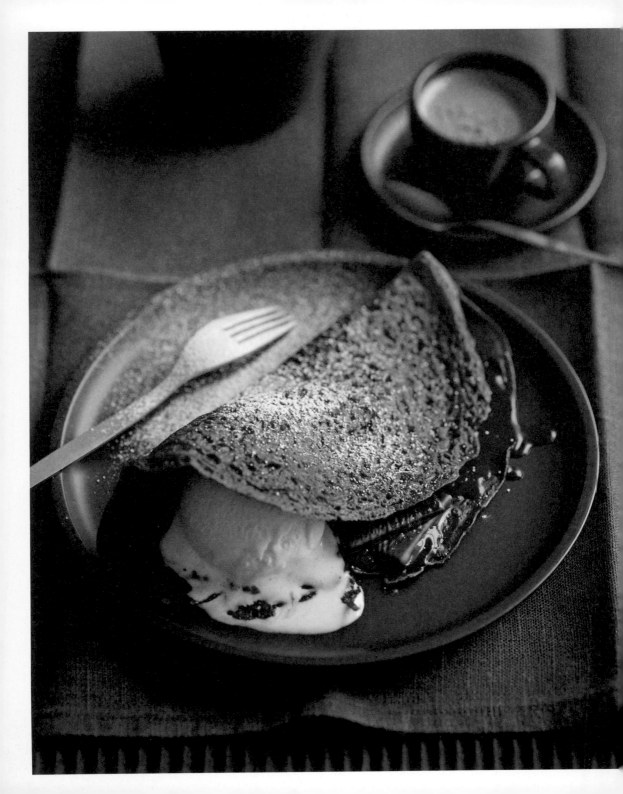

CHOCOLATE MINT CRÊPES

After Eight mints make a rich and indulgent sauce for these crêpes. Serve with a really good-quality vanilla ice cream or mint choc-chip ice cream if you really love peppermint!

PANCAKE BATTER

120 g/1 cup minus 1½ tablespoons plain/all-purpose flour, sifted

30 g/3½ tablespoons cocoa powder

1 egg and 1 egg yolk

2 tablespoons melted butter, cooled, plus extra for frying

15 g/4 teaspoons caster/granulated sugar

pinch of salt

350 ml/1½ cups milk

10 scoops vanilla ice cream or mint choc-chip ice cream, to serve

20 After Eight chocolates or other fondant-filled mints, to serve

icing sugar/confectioners' sugar, to dust

CHOCOLATE MINT SAUCE

200 ml/generous ¾ cup double/heavy cream

150 g/17 After Eight chocolates or other fondant-filled mints

crêpe swizzle stick (optional)

MAKES 10

To make the crêpe batter, put the flour, cocoa powder, egg and egg yolk, melted butter, sugar and salt in a large mixing bowl. Whisking all the time, gradually add the milk until you have a smooth and runny batter. Cover and put the batter in the refrigerator to rest for 30 minutes.

While the batter is resting, make the chocolate mint sauce. Heat the cream and chocolate mints in a saucepan set over a medium heat until the chocolate mints have melted. Keep the pan over a low heat to keep the sauce warm until you are ready to serve.

Remove the batter from the refrigerator and stir gently. Put a little butter in a large frying pan/skillet set over a medium heat. Allow the butter to melt and coat the base of the pan, then ladle a small amount of the rested batter into the pan and quickly spread the batter out very thinly. You can do this either by tilting the pan, or, for best results, use a crêpe swizzle stick. Cook until the top of the pancake is set, then turn it over carefully with a spatula and cook on the other side for a further 1–2 minutes until the crêpe is crispy. Keep the crêpe warm while you cook the remaining batter in the same way.

Place a spoonful or two of the chocolate mint sauce onto each crêpe and top each with a scoop of ice cream and two chocolate mints, then fold the crêpes in half. Dust with icing/confectioners' sugar and serve.

RASPBERRY & CREAM CRÊPES

The tang of fresh raspberries works well with the rich double/heavy cream in these delightful pancakes. Freeze-dried raspberry pieces are available in larger grocery stores or online, but you can omit these if you like.

PANCAKE BATTER

140 g/1 cup plus 1 tablespoon plain/all-purpose flour, sifted

1 egg and 1 egg yolk

2 tablespoons melted butter, cooled, plus extra for frying

15 g/2 teaspoons caster/granulated sugar

pinch of salt

300 ml/1¼ cups whole milk

RASPBERRY SYRUP AND FILLING

800 g/5½ cups fresh raspberries

2 tablespoons icing/confectioners' sugar, sifted

250 ml/1 cup plus 1 tablespoon double/heavy cream, whipped to stiff peaks

handful of freeze-dried raspberry pieces

crêpe swizzle stick (optional)

MAKES 10

Begin by making a raspberry syrup. Press half of the fresh raspberries through a fine meshed sieve/strainer set over a mixing bowl, to release the juice and remove the seeds. Discard the seeds. Add the icing/confectioners' sugar to the raspberry juice and whisk together.

To make the crêpe batter, put the flour, egg and egg yolk, melted butter, caster/granulated sugar and salt in a large mixing bowl. Whisking all the time, gradually add the milk until you have a smooth and runny batter. Add 1 tablespoon of the raspberry syrup and whisk again. Cover and put the batter in the refrigerator to rest for 30 minutes.

While the batter is resting, fold half of the raspberry syrup into the whipped cream so that ripples of syrup run through it. Set aside in the refrigerator until needed.

When you are ready to serve, remove the batter from the refrigerator and stir gently. Put a little butter in a large frying pan/skillet set over a medium heat. Allow the butter to melt and coat the base of the pan, then ladle a small amount of the rested batter into the pan and quickly spread the batter out very thinly. You can do this either by tilting the pan, or, for best results, use a crêpe swizzle stick. Cook until the top of the pancake is set, then turn it over carefully with a spatula and cook on the other side for a further 1–2 minutes until the crêpe is golden brown. Keep the crêpe warm while you cook the remaining batter in the same way.

Spoon some of the raspberry syrup and filling onto one half of each crêpe, then top with a handful of the reserved whole raspberries. Fold each crêpe in half and then in half again.

Sprinkle with freeze-dried raspberries, drizzle with the remaining raspberry syrup and serve.

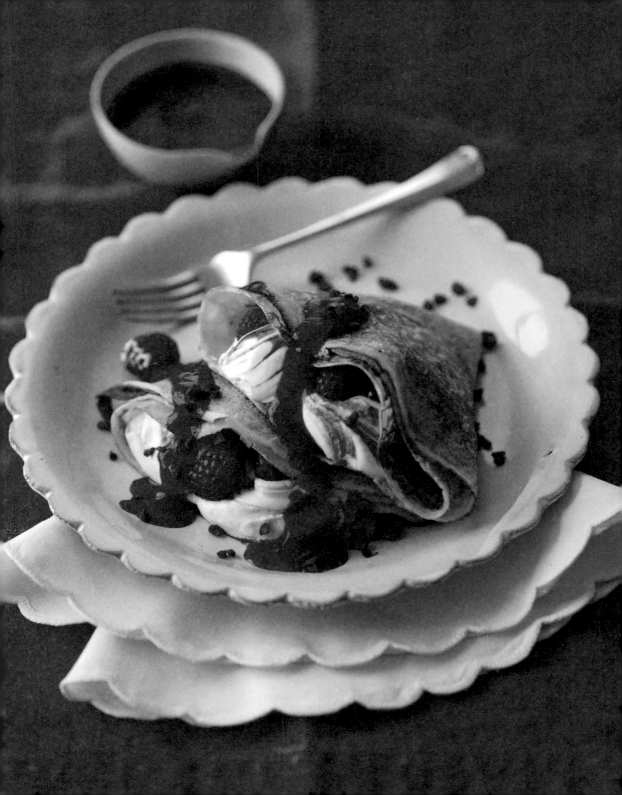

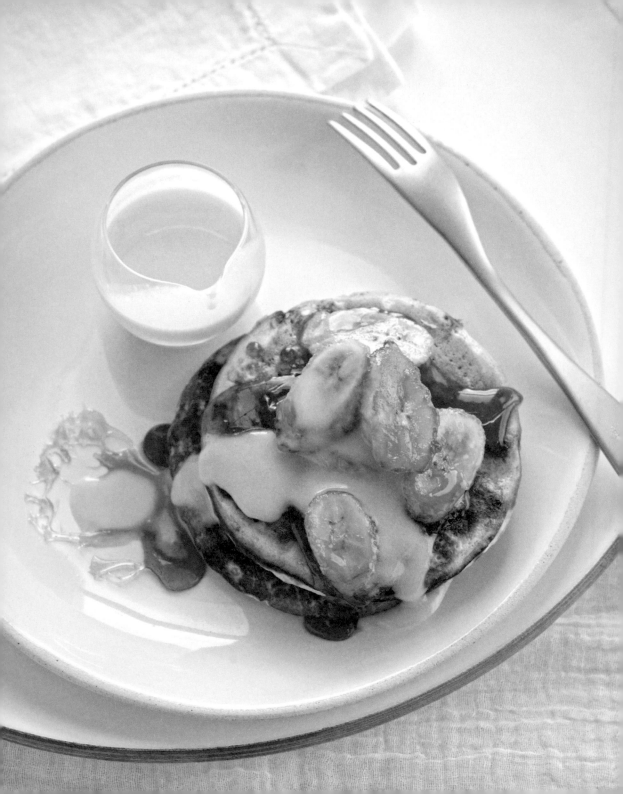

BANANA & CHOC CHIP PANCAKES WITH
MAPLE BUTTER SAUCE & CARAMELIZED BANANAS

PANCAKE BATTER

2 ripe bananas, peeled

freshly squeezed juice of
½ lemon

60 ml/¼ cup maple syrup

pinch of salt

180 g/1⅓ cups self-raising/
rising flour, sifted

1 teaspoon baking powder

1 egg, separated

250 ml/1 cup plus 1 tablespoon
whole milk

3 tablespoons melted butter,
plus extra for frying

100g/⅔ cup milk/semi-sweet
chocolate chips

MAPLE BUTTER SAUCE

50 g/3½ tablespoons butter

80 ml/5 tablespoons maple
syrup

120 ml/½ cup double/
heavy cream

CARAMELIZED BANANAS

4 ripe bananas, peeled and
sliced

2 tablespoons caster/
granulated sugar

MAKES 12

There are few more comforting foods than banana pancakes. These are extra-indulgent, flavoured with maple syrup and bursting with chocolate chips.

Begin by making the pancake batter. Crush the 2 bananas to a smooth purée together with the lemon juice, using a fork or in a food processor. Put the banana purée into a large mixing bowl and add the maple syrup, salt, flour, baking powder and egg yolk. Whisk together the ingredients, gradually adding the milk until the batter is smooth. Whisk in the melted butter. The batter should have a smooth dropping consistency.

In a separate bowl, whisk the egg white to stiff peaks. Gently fold the whisked egg white into the batter together with the chocolate chips using a spatula. Cover and put in the refrigerator to rest for 30 minutes.

Meanwhile, for the sauce, heat the butter and maple syrup in a saucepan set over a medium heat until the butter has melted. Add the cream and simmer over a gentle heat for a few minutes. If you want to serve the sauce warm, keep the pan over the lowest heat until ready to serve.

For the caramelized bananas, coat the banana slices in the sugar all over. Set a frying pan/skillet over a high heat and place the bananas into the dry pan. Cook for a few minutes until the bananas start to caramelize, then turn the slices over and cook on the other side until golden brown. Remove the pan from the heat and set aside.

When you are ready to serve, remove your batter from the refrigerator and stir. Put a little butter in a large frying pan/skillet set over a medium heat. Allow the butter to melt and coat the base of the pan, then ladle small amounts of the batter into the pan, leaving a little space between each. Cook until the underside of each pancake is golden brown and a few bubbles start to appear on the top – this will take about 2–3 minutes. Turn the pancakes over using a spatula and cook on the other side until golden brown. Keep the pancakes warm while you cook the remaining batter in the same way, adding a little butter to the pan each time, if required. Top the pancakes with the caramelized bananas and drizzle with the maple butter sauce to serve.

BLACKBERRY CREAM CHEESE PANCAKES

These pancakes have a hidden pocket of blackberry and cream cheese filling, a yummy surprise when you cut into them! Served with a tangy blackberry sauce and whipped cream, they are an indulgent pancake dessert.

PANCAKE BATTER

160 g/scant 1¼ cups self-raising/rising flour, sifted

1 teaspoon baking powder

1 egg, separated

2 tablespoons caster/granulated sugar

pinch of salt

250 ml/1 cup plus 1 tablespoon whole milk

3 tablespoons melted butter, plus extra for frying

BLACKBERRY SAUCE & FILLING

300 g/2¼ cups fresh blackberries

100 g/½ cup caster/granulated sugar

100 g/½ cup cream cheese

250 ml/1 cup plus 1 tablespoon double/heavy cream, whipped to stiff peaks, to serve

MAKES 6

Begin by making the blackberry sauce and filling. Place the blackberries and sugar in a saucepan with 120 ml/½ cup water over a medium heat, and simmer for about 5 minutes until the fruit is soft and the liquid is syrupy. Leave to cool.

In a separate bowl, whisk together the cream cheese and 2 tablespoons of the cooled blackberries and syrup to make the filling. Refrigerate.

To make the pancake batter, put the flour, baking powder, egg yolk, sugar, salt and milk in a large mixing bowl and whisk together. Whisk in the melted butter. The batter should have a smooth, dropping consistency.

In a separate bowl, whisk the egg white to stiff peaks. Gently fold the whisked egg white into the batter mixture using a spatula. Cover and put in the refrigerator to rest for 30 minutes.

When you are ready to serve, remove your batter mixture from the refrigerator and stir once. Put a little butter in a large frying pan/skillet set over a medium heat. Allow the butter to melt and coat the base of the pan, then ladle some of the batter into the pan and tip to spread the batter out into a circle. Place a spoonful of the blackberry filling in the centre of the pancake and carefully spread it out, leaving a gap between the filling and the edge of the pancake. Cover the filling with a little more pancake batter so that it is completely hidden. Cook until the underside of the pancake is golden brown and a few bubbles start to appear on the top – this will take about 2–3 minutes. Then turn the pancake over using a spatula and cook on the other side until golden brown. Keep the pancake warm while you cook the remaining batter in the same way, adding a little butter to the pan each time, if required.

Serve the pancakes with the reserved blackberry sauce and the whipped cream on the side.

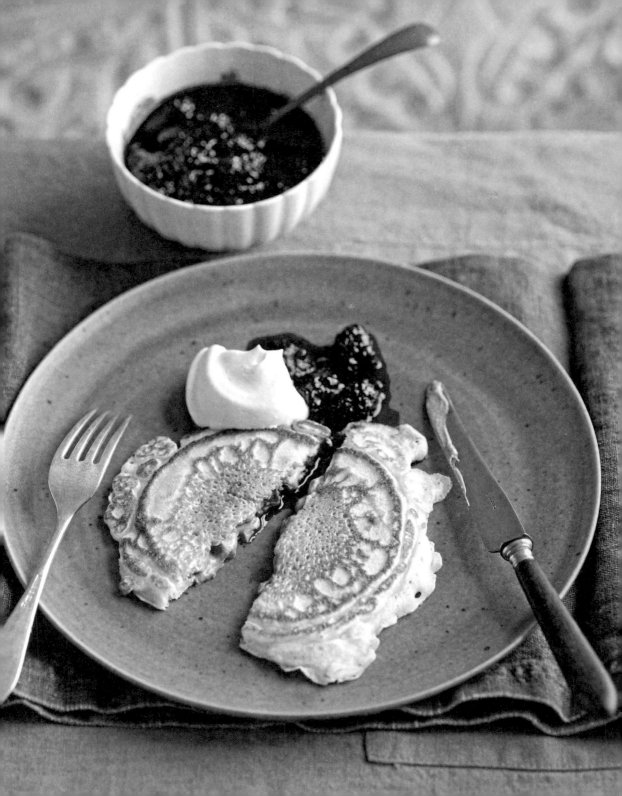

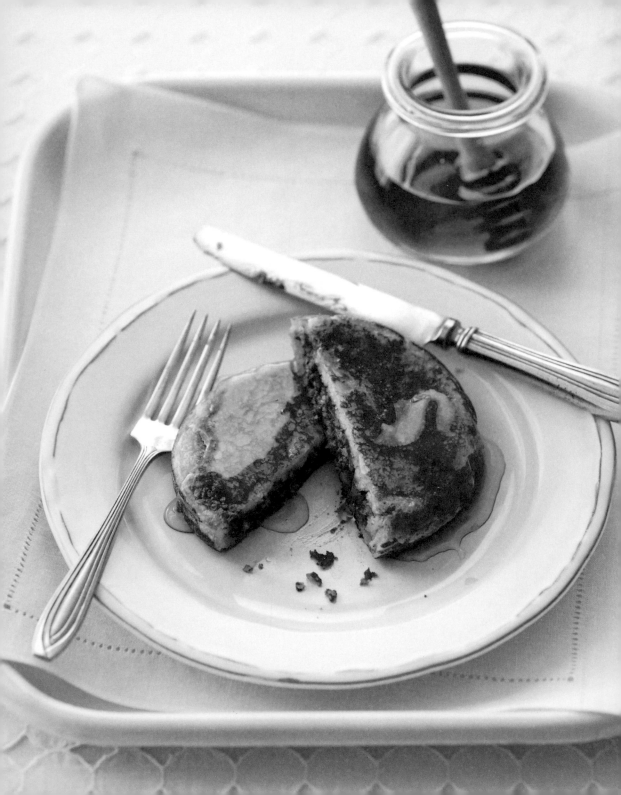

BAKLAVA PANCAKES

Baklava is the utterly delicious Greek sweet treat, with cinnamon and nuts layered between buttery filo/phyllo pastry. The baklava filling inspires these pancakes, which are stuffed with walnut butter and drizzled with honey.

PANCAKE BATTER

160 g/scant 1¼ cups self-raising/rising flour, sifted

1 teaspoon baking powder

1 egg

50 g/¼ cup caster/granulated sugar

½ teaspoon salt

120 ml/½ cup whole milk

280 ml/scant 1¼ cups buttermilk

3 tablespoons melted butter, plus extra for frying

Greek runny honey, to serve

BAKLAVA FILLING

100 g/1 cup chopped walnuts

2 teaspoons ground cinnamon

50 g/¼ cup caster/granulated sugar

90 g/6 tablespoons butter, softened

MAKES 6

To make the pancake batter, put the flour, baking powder, egg, sugar, salt, milk and buttermilk in a large mixing bowl and whisk together. Add the melted butter and whisk again. The batter should have a smooth, pourable consistency. Cover and put in the refrigerator to rest for 30 minutes.

For the baklava filling, blitz the walnuts to a fine crumb with the cinnamon and sugar in a food processor. Transfer to a bowl, then add the butter and mix together to a smooth paste. Set aside.

When you are ready to serve, remove the batter mixture from the refrigerator and stir once. Put a little butter in a large frying pan/skillet set over a medium heat. Allow the butter to melt and coat the base of the pan, then ladle a small amount of the batter into the pan and tip to spread into a small circle. Put a spoonful of the baklava filling in the centre of the pancake and carefully spread it out, leaving a gap between the filling and the edge of the pancake. Cover the filling with a little more pancake batter so that it is completely hidden. Cook until the underside of the pancake is golden brown and a few bubbles start to appear on the top – this will take about 2–3 minutes.

Turn the pancake over using a spatula and cook on the other side until golden brown. Keep the pancake warm while you cook the remaining batter, adding a little butter to the pan each time, if required.

Serve the pancakes warm with a drizzle of honey over the top.

SALTED CARAMEL WAFFLES

If you are a fan of salted caramel, you might find that you could eat this sauce just on its own! But it is delicious with caramel waffles and chocolate curls. The recipe calls for vanilla salt, which is available from delicatessens or online, but if you want to make it yourself then see the Note below.

WAFFLE BATTER

260 g/2 cups self-raising/
   rising flour, sifted

1 teaspoon baking powder

3 eggs, separated

375 ml/1²⁄₃ cups whole milk

75 g/5 tablespoons butter,
   melted, plus extra for
   greasing

50 g/½ cup plain/bittersweet
   chocolate curls, to serve

SALTED CARAMEL SAUCE

150 g/³⁄₄ cup caster/
   granulated sugar

100 g/7 tablespoons butter

1 teaspoon vanilla salt
   (see Note) or sea salt plus
   1 teaspoon vanilla extract

250 ml/1 cup plus 1 tablespoon
   double/heavy cream

*electric or stove-top
   waffle iron*

MAKES 8

Begin by making the salted caramel sauce. Put the sugar and butter in a saucepan set over a medium heat and simmer until both have melted and the resulting caramel starts to turn a deep golden brown colour. Add the vanilla salt and cream and whisk over the heat until the sauce is smooth and glossy. If any lumps of sugar have formed in your sauce, strain through a fine mesh sieve/strainer over a mixing bowl. Set aside to cool.

To make the waffle batter, put the flour, baking powder, egg yolks, milk and melted butter in a large mixing bowl. Whisk until you have a smooth batter. Add 80 ml/scant ⅓ cup of the caramel sauce and whisk again. In a separate mixing bowl, whisk the egg whites to stiff peaks and then gently fold into the batter, a third at a time.

Preheat the waffle iron and grease with a little butter.

Ladle a small amount of the batter into the preheated waffle iron and cook the waffles for 3–5 minutes until golden brown. Keep the waffles warm while you cook the remaining batter in the same way.

Serve the waffles immediately with the caramel sauce on the side, topped with chocolate curls.

Note: To make vanilla salt, split 2 vanilla pods/beans and remove the seeds. Cut the pods in half. Stir the vanilla seeds into several large spoonfuls of sea salt flakes. Place the salt, seeds and vanilla pods/beans in a sterilized airtight jar and set aside for 2 weeks. Discard the vanilla pods/beans before using.

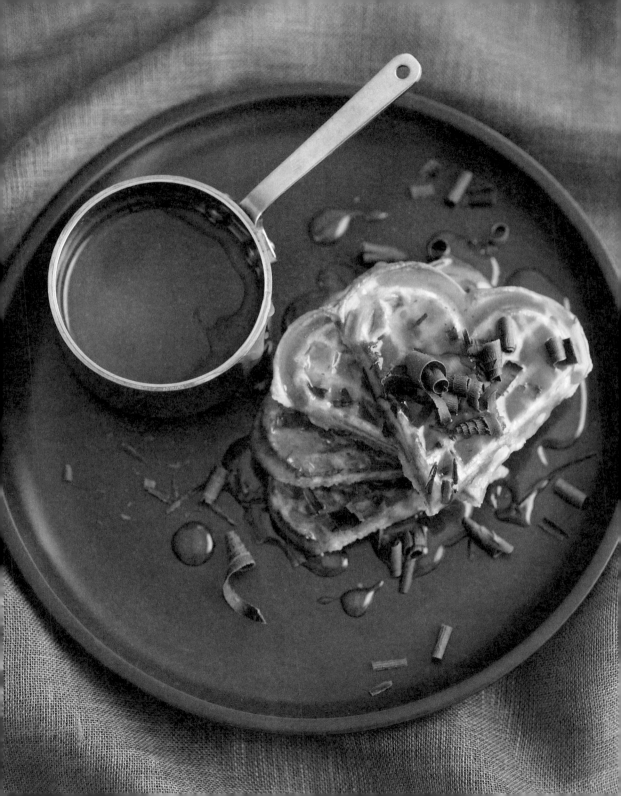

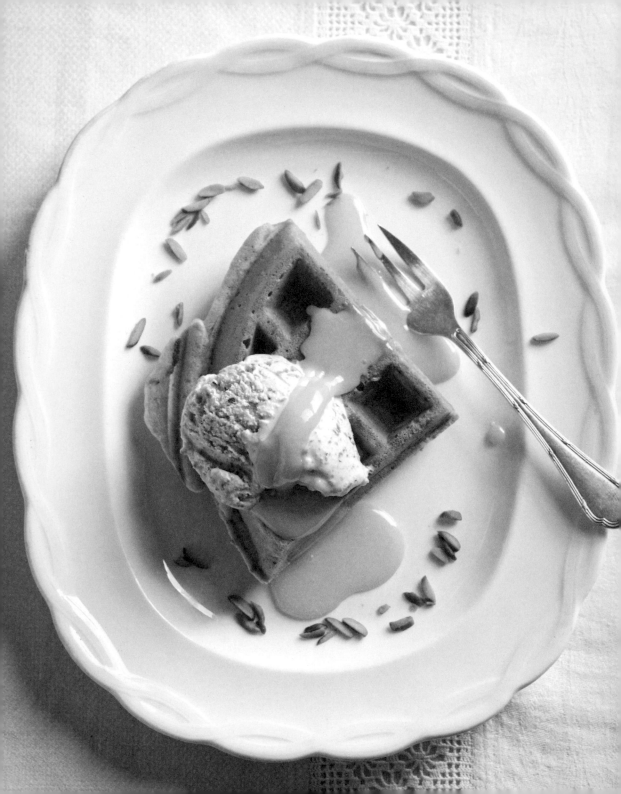

PISTACHIO WAFFLES WITH PISTACHIO ICE CREAM & WHITE CHOCOLATE SAUCE

Pistachio ice cream has a delicate, perfumed flavour and is a great accompaniment to these nutty waffles drenched in heavenly white chocolate sauce. If you are short of time, you could use store-bought ice cream instead.

WAFFLE BATTER

100 g/¾ cup pistachios, plus a handful finely chopped, to decorate

240 g/1¾ cups self-raising/ rising flour, sifted

60 g/scant ⅓ cup caster/ granulated sugar

pinch of salt

3 eggs, separated

375 ml/1⅔ cups whole milk

4 tablespoons butter, melted, plus extra for greasing

ICE CREAM

100 g/¾ cup pistachios

400 ml/1¾ cups double/ heavy cream

200 ml/generous ¾ cup milk

5 egg yolks

100 g/½ cup caster/ granulated sugar

WHITE CHOCOLATE SAUCE

200 g/1⅓ cups white chocolate

250 ml/1 cup plus 1 tablespoon double/heavy cream

electric or stove-top waffle iron

ice-cream machine (optional)

MAKES 8

Begin by preparing the ice cream. Put the pistachios in a food processor and pulse to a fine crumb. Transfer the finely ground pistachios to a saucepan set over a high heat together with the double/heavy cream and milk. Bring the mixture to the boil, then remove from the heat and leave to infuse for 30 minutes. In a mixing bowl, whisk together the egg yolks and sugar until very thick and pale yellow. Return the pistachio milk to the heat and bring to the boil again. Pour the boiling pistachio milk over the eggs in a thin stream, whisking all the time. Return the mixture to the pan and cook for a few minutes longer until it begins to thicken. Leave to cool completely. Churn in an ice-cream machine following the manufacturer's instructions. Transfer to a freezer proof container and store in the freezer until you are ready to serve.

For the sauce, put the white chocolate and double/heavy cream in a saucepan or pot set over a medium heat and simmer until the chocolate has melted, stirring all the time. Keep the pan on the heat but turn it down to low to keep the sauce warm until you are ready to serve.

To make the waffle batter, put the pistachios in a food processor and pulse to a fine crumb. Place the pistachios in a large mixing bowl with the flour, sugar, salt, egg yolks, milk and melted butter. Whisk until you have a smooth batter. In a separate mixing bowl, whisk the egg whites to stiff peaks and then gently fold into the batter, a third at a time.

Preheat the waffle iron and grease with a little butter.

Ladle a small amount of the batter into the preheated waffle iron and cook the waffles for 2–3 minutes until golden brown. Keep the waffles warm while you cook the remaining batter in the same way.

Serve the waffles topped with generous scoops of ice cream and drizzled with the white chocolate sauce. Decorate with the chopped pistachios.

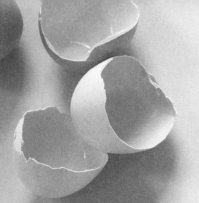

RED VELVET CRÊPE CAKE

Ideal for a birthday or special celebration, why not whip up this show-stopping cake for that pancake-obsessed friend or family member in your life?

vegetable oil spray

1 tablespoon pink heart-shaped sprinkles

PANCAKE BATTER

150 g/generous 1 cup plain/ all-purpose flour, sifted

3 tablespoons cocoa powder

pinch of salt

50 g/¼ cup caster/superfine sugar

3 eggs, beaten

250 ml/1 cup plus 1 tablespoon whole milk

150 ml/⅔ cup sour/soured cream

1 tablespoon vanilla extract

red gel or paste food colouring

CREAM CHEESE FILLING

375 g/2⅔ cups icing/ confectioners' sugar, sifted

750 g/3⅓ cups full-fat cream cheese

17-cm/6¾-inch frying pan/ skillet

disposable piping/pastry bag fitted with a large star nozzle/tip

SERVES 20

For the pancake batter, mix the dry ingredients together in a bowl, then create a well in the centre. Mix the wet ingredients together in a jug/pitcher (except the food colouring) and gradually pour into the well, gently whisking to mix the wet and dry ingredients together. Stir through enough red food colouring to get a mid-bright shade.

Spray the frying pan/skillet with the oil spray and heat over a medium heat. Add a small ladleful of the batter to the pan. Tilt the pan so the batter covers the base and then cook for around 30–60 seconds until cooked underneath. Flip or turn the pancake and cook for another 30–60 seconds. Remove to a wire rack, then re-spray the pan with the oil spray and repeat. You should get around 20 pancakes. Allow to cool.

For the filling, beat the icing/confectioners' sugar into the cream cheese, in manageable batches, with an electric hand whisk until smooth. Put 150 g/5½ oz. of the mixture into a small bowl, cover and chill whilst you use the remaining filling to stack the pancakes.

Stack the pancakes with a layer of the cream cheese filling between each. Fill the piping/pastry bag fitted with a large star nozzle/tip with the reserved chilled filling and pipe small star-shaped blobs around the top edge. Scatter with the sprinkles. Chill in the refrigerator for at least 2 hours before serving.

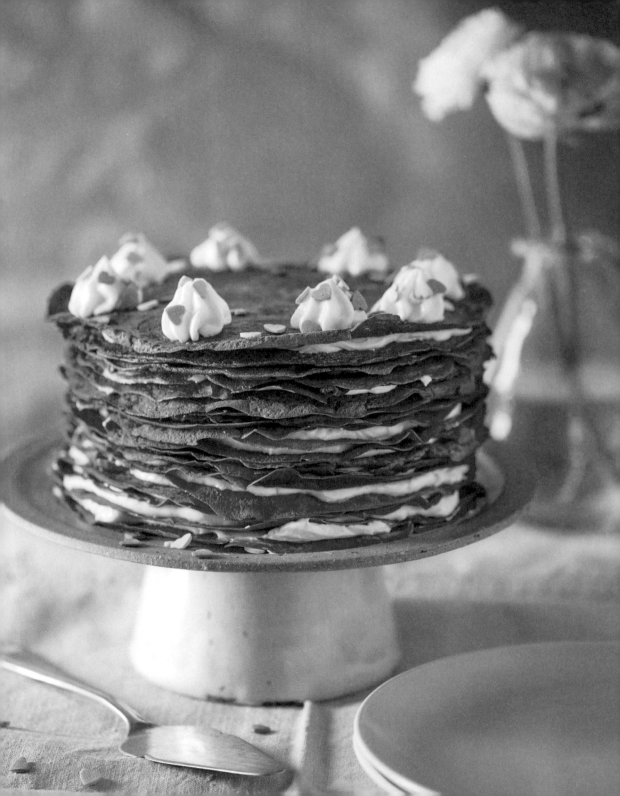

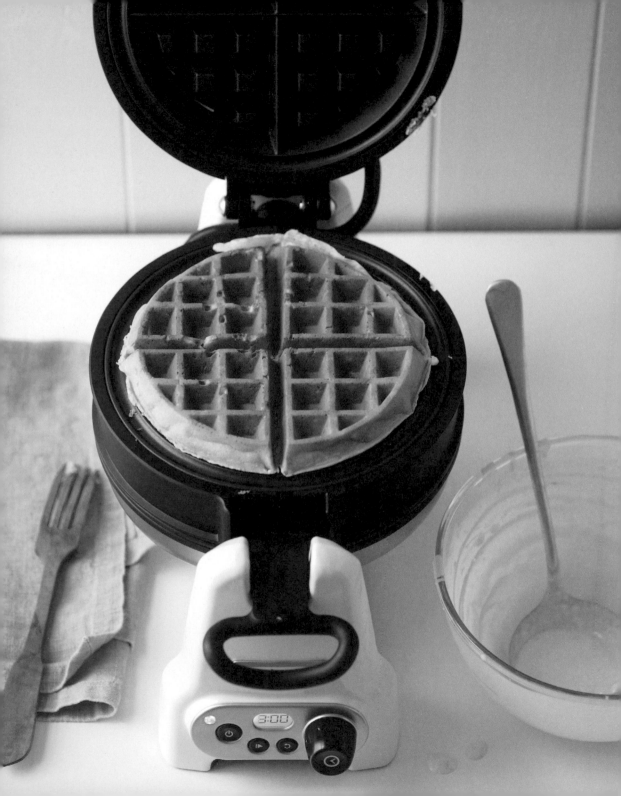